D0968946

"Cookie has written a book that can ch [...] what it teaches. Losing weight does n[...] frustration and hate. She shows you t[...] curiosity and wonder that reveals the reasons you are overeating and not living at your ideal weight. Once you discover why, the 'how to change' becomes so much easier. Your best tool for losing weight is your mind, and "Clearing Your Path to Permanent Weight Loss" shows you how to use it."

~Brooke Castillo, author of *If I Am So Smart, Why Can't I Lose Weight?*

"Cookie Rosenblum's book, *Clearing Your Path to Permanent Weight Loss*, is a wonderful guide for anyone who is tired of dieting, and looking for a fresh perspective on lasting weight loss. Rosenblum is empathetic yet empowering, supportive yet stirring; and her book will get you out of your comfort zone and moving toward bold - yet real and achievable - weight loss goals. This isn't a diet book, and Rosenblum will help you understand *why* going on another restrictive diet is definitely *not* the solution. Through a series of intuitive worksheets throughout the book, you will discover why your previous weight loss efforts have failed, and you will create your own path toward success. The author helps you target your destructive thought processes, while helping you shift your focus to your strengths and what will help you change now. You will learn to look at your weight loss challenge in the most positive, practical light, and begin using loving self-discipline. You'll learn to make genuine choices that fit your life, and aim for the weight loss results that are right for *you* – not a movie star, and not your inner perfectionist. I highly recommend this book to anyone struggling to lose weight for good."

~Kathryn Hansen, author of *Brain over Binge: Why I Was Bulimic, Why Conventional Therapy Didn't Work and How I Recovered for Good.*

"If you've ever wished for someone who can teach you to lose and maintain weight without struggle, your wish has been granted. Cookie Rosenblum's compassion, information, and experience can unravel the tangle of anxiety and compulsion around food and weight, teaching you to think and behave like one of those naturally thin people you've envied for years. A fabulous Cookie that actually makes you fit—dreams really do come true!"

~Martha Beck, Life Coach, Columnist, and Author, about Cookie Rosenblum

"*Clearing Your Path to Permanent Weight Loss* provides a fantastic guide for moving past the roadblocks that get in the way of long-term change. This book is a wonderful resource for anyone who is stuck and not making progress. It shows you how to get beyond past failures and find true weight-loss success."

~Linda Spangle, RN, MA, author of *Life is Hard, Food is Easy* and *100 Days of Weight Loss*

"Cookie has written a compelling and compassionate book to help end your weight loss struggle. It's also a book about the hope and self-love required to take a leap of faith into the world of permanent health. If you are ready to shed the old and build something new, dive in!"

~Susan Hyatt, Author, TV Show Host and Master Certified Life Coach, author of *Create Your Own Luck: 7 Steps to Get Your Lucky On*

"Cookie Rosenblum is an insightful and compassionate weight loss coach. Her understanding of how the brain works and how life works gives her a valuable edge in guiding you through the journey from diet obsession to personal freedom about food and weight. Her new book is filled with practical exercises that make it quick and easy to implement her valuable coaching expertise. It's a down-to-earth and real-speak book that offers not just weight loss suggestions but helps you make the important connections to your own life that are the key to true understanding and real differences in the way you eat, think and live."

~Lori Dube, MSW

"Cookie Rosenblum draws on her many years as a successful weight loss coach, to help you change your relationship with food by changing your mindset. No more white-knuckling your way through deprivation and micro-managed eating. Her wisdom and tools will help you approach weight loss from the inside out - from a place of peace, self-acceptance, and compassion. She will guide you as you clear your path to not just lose the weight, but to lose the whole problem."

~Kay Duncan, LICSW, Psychotherapist and Eating Disorders Specialist. Bellevue, WA

Clearing Your Path to Permanent Weight Loss

The truth about why you've failed in the past, and what you *must* know to succeed now

By Cookie Rosenblum, M.A.

Printed in the United States of America

First Printing, 2014

ISBN-10: 099139190X

ISBN-13: 978-0-9913919-0-5

Published by Real Weight Loss for Real Women

RealWeightLossRealWomen.com

Cover design by Kimb Manson Graphic Design

Interior formatting and design by The Eyes for Editing

For David, Sara and Sophia,

whose presence in my life

reminds me of what is important, every day.

And for all my family, friends, coaches and clients, who

have contributed to my life, my work, and this book

in ways I cannot count.

Table of Contents

Introduction: Why I Wrote This Book

I've been a weight loss coach since 1986. During the course of those years, I've coached many, many women on how to lose weight. They come to me feeling defeated, battered, and unworthy.

Many of them think something must be wrong with them.

Here are some of the things I've heard:

How can I run a company but not be in charge of my own body?

What is wrong with me that I can't stick to any weight loss plan?

So many things in my life are going well... I just can't believe that I can't master this one thing!

I'm so frustrated. I feel like giving up... but I know I'm smart, and I see other women succeeding at weight loss. What is my problem?

Most women express some version of these thoughts when they come to work with me after trying many different weight loss plans. The problem is they keep repeating the same actions over and over again... and guess what? Of course! They get the same results.

They keep repeating the same actions because they haven't cleared up what's blocking them in the first place.

If you don't know why you're overeating, no diet book or plan or guru will help you lose weight.

Or if you do, it will be temporary, only to bounce back on as soon as you go back to living the life you've been living.

And if you've tried countless times to lose your extra weight but can't, you are probably not clear about *why* nothing has worked for you.

Something has to give.

So, I wrote this book.

To teach you how to be different.

How to be one of the ones who succeed.

And here's the thing—it's not about being successful at eating less and exercising more.

It's about getting to the root of the problem... and finally finding out, on a deep level, why you turn to food when you aren't hungry.

You may think it's because something just tastes good.

It's not.

You may think it's because you need to eat to get through a difficult time and after that, you'll get really, really strict with yourself.

It's not.

Or, you may think maybe you just haven't found the magical plan that will give you that perfect body you see in the magazines.

It's not.

So, what is it about?

It's about first, clearing your path. Figuring out what you've been doing and why.

It's about seeing your patterns.

Learning from the times you fell down.

And understanding why you go to food in the first place when you aren't hungry.

Look, when you want to accomplish something big, and permanent weight loss is really big, you need to prepare.

You need to slow down and take a look at yourself.

Get all the details of who you are, why you want this, and what's held you back up to this point.

Then, systematically, you learn to deal with what went wrong in the past.

Not to dwell on it. But to correct it.

Every single thing we do comes from the way we think. Seriously. As humans, we don't take any action without having a thought first. So if there are women in the world who are at their natural weight without dieting, we need to look at the way they think. And learn from them.

This book is an offering to you.

To help you take the first steps toward creating a body that looks and feels good.

And that starts from the inside.

In your head.

In your thoughts to be exact.

What we will do together is explore what you've been through, help you get some answers, and then feel good enough to begin to lose weight from a place of peace.

Without hating yourself.

Without desperation.

And certainly not in frustration.

Those feelings just won't get you there.

You've tried.

I've tried.

And most of my clients tried.

Those lousy feelings don't work to give you what you want. Freedom from obsessing about your weight, and what you eat, and how you look.

Here is what does work: taking a deep look at yourself and how you got to this point. Then, taking the time to understand why you've failed. And finally, learning the tools that will get you ready to roll. And give you what you want most.

Permanent weight loss. So you don't just lose the weight, you lose the whole problem!

Here's how to do this. Create some time and space in your

day to read one lesson at a time. And then dive deeper and do the corresponding worksheet.

Get to know yourself.

Discover your strengths and your challenges.

Learn how to use these strengths to overcome your challenges *so when you make an effort to change your habits and thoughts and behaviors, you will be armed and ready.*

When you take the time to do these worksheets, you are personalizing the lessons. You aren't just reading words in a book, but thinking and internalizing what you learn.

These lessons will uncover whatever has prevented you from achieving your dream of lasting weight loss.

When we read something, we think about it briefly. We notice things that feel right to us. But when we take the next step and write about how we can live what we've read, we can change on a whole new level. And that's what you want.

These lessons and worksheets have helped so many of my clients conquer their weight issues. And I know they can help you, too.

I'm so proud of you for doing this work, and I hope you feel proud of yourself.

Enjoy, and don't forget to email me with any questions you have. I'm here to help you on this journey. (cookie@RealWeightLossRealWomen.com)

xoxo, Cookie

What Went Wrong?

Did you take a look at why you didn't succeed?

You didn't take the time to sit down and figure out why your past weight loss efforts didn't work. You feel bad and blame yourself. But you're not analyzing *exactly what happened*.

Lesson 1: Why You Need to Clear Your Path

Here's our focus for today: Learn why it's critical to clear your path of past mistakes so you can move toward permanent weight loss.

You want to lose weight.

You've found a program that sounds good.

Before you take that leap, take a moment and consider this:

You need to slow down long enough to think about where you are right now, and why you are there.

If you don't, you are bound to repeat the same errors you've always made. And we both know what that will give you: the same results you've always gotten.

So in order to lose your extra weight once and for all, let's spend a few minutes together each day and take a look at what has gone wrong in the past... so it will go well for you in the future.

I'd like you to think loosely about why your weight loss efforts haven't worked so far... or maybe they've worked, but haven't lasted.

Are there some obvious patterns that you know you keep repeating?

In the coming days, we'll look closely at these patterns. For right now, just know this: **your past errors were not a waste of time. They serve to show you exactly what needs to change as you move forward.** They will be lessons that are invaluable, and will help you on your journey toward lasting weight loss.

When we're trying to accomplish a big goal like weight loss, roadblocks will come up. You are stretching yourself to do something different for you, out of the box. Well, when you do this, part of the process is that your fears, your mental blocks, and your habits will all come up.

What I'd like you to see is that these road blocks are merely learning points. If you don't stop and review them and make some changes, you are destined to repeat them... no matter what eating plan you follow.

I'd like you to take a leap here and see yourself as a woman who is learning as she grows... In fact, falling down while you learn is absolutely part of the growth process. Imagine how babies learn to walk. They crawl, they stand up, and they fall down. Then they keep getting back up. If they didn't keep getting back up, they wouldn't strengthen their leg muscles enough for walking. The very act of falling down and pulling themselves up each time makes them strong enough to eventually walk.

And so it is with you, too.

You keep trying and falling down.

You almost give up. And then your desire to try again is stronger than your fear of failing. So you give it another try.

This is good stuff.

As long as you learn from your falls. And that's exactly what we are going to do here.

All I ask is that you give yourself ten or fifteen minutes a day to read and think about your daily lesson. If you'd like to learn on an even deeper level, go to the corresponding worksheet and do the written exercise. Give it to yourself as a gift.

Where you are now is exactly where you are meant to be.

Allow yourself right now to reach a place of peacefulness so you can get up again and move forward. With new knowledge and self-love.

I'll be right here with you.

Dive deeper into this concept. Go to the corresponding worksheet and do the exercise.

Worksheet 1: Clear Your Path

All of the things we tell ourselves, whether we're aware of them or not, have a great influence on our actions. So if on the surface we're thinking we can handle something, but on the inside, we're thinking "No way... I can't do this," guess which side wins? The inside voice that you may not even be conscious of *will always win.*

That's why we are embarking on this journey of clearing your path so you can begin to lose weight.

Start by listing all the reasons you think you *can't* do this.

What is "wrong" with you?

Why will you fail again?

Let's just get those reasons out of your head, so we can release them and move on. Think of this as a giant download.

List and release... nothing will be left lurking in there to sabotage you. I promise we will deal with all these thoughts soon. But for now, just clean up your thinking and get them out.

Reasons I believe I haven't been able to lose weight: /maintain weight loss

1. I'm not strong enough
2. It's just a bite
3. I can handle having a wide variety of foods
4. Hormones
5. Stress
6. Bad marriage (when I was married)
7. Everyone in my family is fat, so I will be too
8. It's too hard
9. I'm not disciplined enough
10. I'm not strong enough

What Went Wrong?

Do you still think there's a magical diet out there?

You still hold onto the hope that there is some diet out there that will work for you. You think you just haven't found the magical answer yet.

Lesson 2: Understand, Once and for All, Why Diets Aren't the Answer

You've heard the expression "diets don't work" about 7,293 times.

I know that *you* know it's true.

> *We cannot solve our problems with the same level of thinking that created them.*
>
> ~Albert Einstein

In your vast experience and experimentation, you've gathered great evidence that proves that diets don't work.

And yet.

Your ears still perk up when someone mentions a weight loss plan they just heard about.

Because secretly, you still hope there is some method, some book, some program, or some guru who possesses the answer.

So I want to give you a clear and definitive perspective about why diets don't work for weight loss.

In the past 70 years, lots of research has been done looking at various weight loss methods.

And the research shows that dieting and the restriction that goes with it does not lead to weight loss.

In fact, it actually leads to weight gain. And frequently to binge eating!

Dieting to lose weight simply is not effective.

In 2007, a team from UCLA analyzed all long-term diet studies ever published up to that date[1].

The results showed conclusively that only a minute percentage of people lost a small percentage of their weight.

And they almost always gained it back.

In fact, most regained the weight plus some extra weight.

They also found that dieting was the best predictor of future weight gain!

So even though you hate your extra weight and would do almost anything to get rid of it, the method (diets) you've chosen to get rid of it simply doesn't work.

And in the long run, it will give you the exact opposite result you want!

To lose weight, you need to stop dieting, get to the reason you are overeating, and deal with it.

---

1 The UCLA research: http://newsroom.ucla.edu/portal/ucla/dieting-does-not-work-ucla-researchers-7832.aspx

That's it.

Stop wasting your precious time and energy looking for the secret, new solution. Let's start looking at the reasons you're eating more than your body needs, and go from there.

Dive deeper into this concept. Go to the corresponding worksheet and do the exercise.

Worksheet 2: Kiss Diets of the Past Good-bye

Looking back at your dieting history, I'll bet that you've tried or at least considered some "interesting" diets.

Some sound so strange we might not like to admit they're on our list. Remember the banana diet?

And some sound so reasonable we were perplexed that we *couldn't* make them work.

Now we know for sure that no matter what the diet entailed, it was doomed to fail. It's not us at all. It's simply the fact that restricting our food stimulates our brain's survival mechanism, causing us to overeat and gain weight.

Let's have a proper farewell and burial for all diets past:

1. What diet did you try or think about trying?

The south Beach Diet, the virgin
Diet, food restriction, intermittant
fasting, low carb

2. What happened?

For many of them, I gained the weight back, or — as I am currently (c int. fasting), began binging and /or overeating

3. Can you kiss it good-bye peacefully?

Yes. Goodbye damn diets!

Repeat this process for every diet you can remember. Let's officially get them out of our systems, our memories, and our lives. And make room for what *does* work.

What Went Wrong?

Do you hate your weight so much that you can't move forward?

You are *overly focused on how much you weigh,* and you are making it mean painful things about yourself. This makes you feel terrible, which makes you overeat even more.

Lesson 3: Start Here: Pick a Number, Any Number

Today's focus will be on not letting the number on your scale today mean anything that will hold you back on this journey.

You are not your weight! Why am I saying this so strongly to you?

Because of the misguided way so many of us use our body weight number.

We tend to use that number to beat ourselves with.

What do I mean?

What we weigh is simply a number. It's a number on a piece of metal and plastic... your infamous scale.

This number reflects the amount of blood, tissue, fluid and bone you have in your body at this moment. It will change when you drink a cup of coffee. Or go to the bathroom. Or have lunch.

On any given day, this number is a fleeting reflection of something physical. It has nothing to do with who you are as a person. Whether you've been good or bad, whether you've failed or succeeded. And yet many of us have a tendency to punish ourselves because of this number.

And, here's the kicker... when we're finished beating ourselves, we feel so bad we want to go eat something so we can escape that bad feeling.

What a crazy cycle!

In order to move ahead on this weight loss journey, we need to stop making our scale number mean anything more than it does.

It has no bearing on how smart we are.

It has no bearing on our future successes in any area of life.

And it really has no bearing on our future weight loss achievements.

But, using it as a weapon does have an effect on us...a very, very negative effect. We simply can't get where we want to go while flogging ourselves with our "terrible" number.

The way to continue on this journey is to level the playing field and start from a place of acceptance. Hating ourselves because we don't like our weight puts us at a distinct disadvantage. But if we can go on this trip with love and acceptance, we can learn from the past and move peacefully into our future.

We are complicated creatures. Our body weight is a miniscule part of our self-description.

Look at your current weight as your starting place.

Drop the hate and anger.

Wherever you are is a great place to start.

Dive deeper into this concept. Go to the corresponding worksheet and do the exercise.

Worksheet 3: Start Here with Whatever You Weigh

Ah, the dreaded scale. Our goal here is to take away the bad feelings we get when we get on the scale and see a number that we don't like. First, know that all numbers on the scale are neutral. There is no such thing as a bad number. When you get on the scale, the number you see means, "this is my starting place" If you get any bad feelings on the scale, it's simply because of what you're telling yourself.

So I'd like you to weigh yourself three days in a row.

Look at the number and fill out the questions below. **You are not allowed to beat yourself!** Seriously, in order to move forward, I want you to see what comes up when you see your number. Notice it and *see if you can think of the scale number in a more neutral way.* An example might be:

Number: 187

Thought: I'm so fat! What's wrong with me?

New thought: 187, that's a great place to start. Or, 187, I'm in the process of getting to a lower weight.

Your turn:

1. Your number: 138.

4/ /2022

Thought: Yes!. This is a pretty low number for me. I'm finally skinny.

New thought: This is a good place to start. I'm in the process of still losing and & maintaining my weight.

2. Your number:

4| |2022 **Thought:**_____

_____

_____

_____

New thought:_____

_____

_____

_____

3. Your number:_

4| |2022 **Thought:**_____

_____

_____

_____

New thought:_____

_____

_____

_____

What Went Wrong?

Are you afraid you'll never change if you learn to accept yourself?

You hear about self-acceptance, but you're afraid that if you try it, you'll never change or lose weight.

Lesson 4: Self-acceptance Does Not Equal Self-indulgence

Today's lesson is all about how to accept yourself now without fearing that self-acceptance means giving in to self-indulgence.

So, I'm advising you to be compassionate and accepting of yourself in order to move on in your journey.

But I can just hear you now: doesn't accepting myself as I am right now mean that I'll never lose weight? That I'll never reach my goals? That I'll never get up off the couch?

Do you believe that self-acceptance means that you will lie on a couch all day and eat chocolates?

Sorry. Let's clear this up so you can continue to move forward.

There's a big difference between self-acceptance and self-indulgence.

Self-acceptance means that you can embrace who you are. With some extra weight. And wrinkles, and sags and rolls. And gray hair and breakouts and sun spots.

Oh my. Why would you want to do that?

Because it's hard, no, actually it's impossible to put yourself out there and ask for love from the world when you can't muster it up for yourself.

> *I'm hard on myself, so I'm working on shifting perspective toward self-acceptance, with all my flaws and weaknesses*
>
> ~Gwyneth Paltrow

Self-acceptance is an inside job that paves the way for the world to fall in love with you.

And there is no trick you can employ that will let you skip this step.

And by the way, if you choose to not accept yourself right now, you are essentially rejecting yourself!

Does that change your weight? NO. It just feels bad.

Start slowly by noticing little things that make you unique and that you can LEARN to appreciate. Be gentle with yourself. Notice a flaw and smile about it. It's a part of you. Yes, you can still learn to change it. But first you need to accept it.

And how does this relate to self-indulgence?

You wouldn't believe the number of clients I work

with who are terribly afraid that if they break down and accept themselves as they are that this means they will never change.

Never move forward.

And certainly never lose weight.

Oh no. They envision themselves lying around, eating junk food, and being unproductive and disconnected.

Sorry to bust this myth, but I'm here to tell you that you need to let go of this belief.

Here's what self-indulgence really looks like:

Self-indulgence means that you allow yourself to do whatever you want in the moment with no concern about consequences at all. Like a child.

Self-indulgence is actually very childlike behavior. It means we bring out our inner brat, who wants everything and wants it now. Who could care less about consequences. Who wants results that don't come from their behavior.

To tell you the truth, self-indulgence on an everyday basis doesn't really feel as good as we think it will. Giving ourselves what we want in the moment feels great... for that moment. But if we indulge in overeating, overdrinking, or overspending on a regular basis, we are satisfying the urge of the minute and we will pay for it down the road. How? By creating results we don't really want.

What really works better is self-discipline.

Now, wait, just a minute.

I'm not talking about cracking the whip on yourself and being strict and punishing.

No one wants that.

I'm talking about looking at self-discipline as a reflection of how much you love yourself and want the best for yourself.

It's about getting yourself to do what is in your best interest.

It's about taking yourself by the hand and going to bed when you're tired. Feeding yourself when you're hungry. Giving yourself quality food. And rest time. And high-quality connections.

Because you deserve it.

And this takes discipline. Because sometimes, in the moment, we tell ourselves that it's easier to go for the junk.

So, self-acceptance comes first. And loving self-discipline will help you get there. And if you work on these two things, I don't think I'll find you cemented to your couch eating potato chips.

Dive deeper into this concept. Go to the corresponding worksheet and do the exercise.

Worksheet 4: Self-acceptance Leading to Change

Self-acceptance means you care for and accept yourself right now. No matter what you weigh. And **self-indulgence means giving yourself whatever you want, whenever you want it, with no regard for what is *really* best for you.**

Two pretty different concepts, right?

Our goal is to be self-accepting, so we can feel peace and contentment and move on with our goals. When we accept ourselves in a loving way, it paves the way for us to grow. Many of us think if we accept ourselves, we will stay just the way we are... This is definitely not true. Hatred, disgust, and force don't make us change, but **self-acceptance allows change.**

Think of something you'd like to change about yourself. Now think of where you are right now, related to this thing you'd like to change. Take a breath and get quiet.

25

And now just accept where you are. No arguments, no buts. Just thoughts like: **this is where I am right now, and that's okay.**

This is where I am right now. I both overate and binge-ate today. But its oc. I'm ok.

Now think of a time when you were trying to be "good" to yourself and you ended up being self-indulgent. What did you do? Did it really feel good after the moment wore off?

I overate, massively. No. It did not feel good. I kicked myself the whole rest of the day.

What Went Wrong?

Do you think of your extra weight as your fault?

You don't own the fact that your **actions created your current weight**. You need to take responsibility for your weight. But you just can't seem to do this *without beating yourself up*.

Lesson 5: Taking Responsibility for Your Weight without Beating Yourself Up

---

Your focus for today is learning how to take responsibility for your current weight, with compassion.

Let's assume, for a moment, that you are X pounds overweight. This extra weight doesn't feel good *or* natural to you and you want to get it off. Right now. In fact, you would have liked it to be off yesterday.

And you are mad at yourself for putting it on in the first place.

How do you get out of this circular thinking where you know what you want, but you just keep going around blaming yourself for being here now?

First, own it. Own your weight. Accept responsibility for whatever your number is today.

How, you may ask? I'm so mad at myself for overeating, again!

Your extra weight is a result of your actions. You may have eaten when you weren't hungry. You may have kept eating way past being satisfied. Or you may have used food to temporarily feel better when you were upset.

It doesn't matter how this extra weight came about. What matters is your willingness to acknowledge that you created it. You made choices and acted in a way that allowed your body to store extra calories.

Your second step is to sit with the responsibility for your weight, but at the same time, to be compassionate toward yourself.

The way to take responsibility for your current weight without beating yourself up is this thought: **You did the best you could at that time to care for yourself.** Was extra food a great way to care for you? Clearly not. But it was the best you were capable of at the time.

And here's some good news: **if you created this weight because of your actions, then you're totally capable of creating something different**. And that's exactly what you will do after you clear away all these roadblocks.

Forgiving yourself for where you are takes away blame and judgment.

Both blame and judgment keep you stuck, right where you DON"T want to be: overweight and feeling terrible and blaming yourself!

When we call ourselves nasty names, the only thing it accomplishes is making us feel awful.

And when we can allow ourselves to feel compassion,

we're giving ourselves a great gift: clearance to move ahead and take steps to get to the heart of our weight issues.

Give yourself this gift.

It doesn't mean you won't move ahead.

It means you will move ahead easier. Without the self-beating. It will feel so much better!

Dive deeper into this concept. Go to the corresponding worksheet and do the exercise.

Worksheet 5: Taking Responsibility with Compassion

Of course you should take complete responsibility for yourself. For all the actions you have taken that have brought you to where you are now. But there is **no benefit** to taking responsibility and then beating yourself. That has to stop right here.

Your goal is to take responsibility for your current results **with** compassion. A good way to think about this is to imagine you are talking to a beloved friend. She is confessing her transgressions and errors to you. How would you respond?

Your harsh thought: I can't stick to any program for longer than a week. I have no willpower.

Your compassionate response: I've done many things in my life for longer than a week. I just need to find a different way to look at this.

This does not mean that you're making excuses for yourself. It simply means that you will move forward more with love than with self-hatred.

Go back to Lesson 1 and list some of the thoughts you downloaded about yourself. Painful thoughts. Now see if you can come up with a compassionate response, just as you would for someone you love.

1. Your harsh thought:_____

_____

_____

_____

Your compassionate response:_____

_____

_____

_____

2. Your harsh thought:_____

_____

_____

_____

Your compassionate response: _____

_____

_____

_____

3. Your harsh thought:_____

_____

_____

_____

Your compassionate response:_____

_____

_____

_____

4. Your harsh thought:_____

_____

_____

_____

Your compassionate response:_____

_____

_____

_____

5. Your harsh thought:_____

_____

_____

_____

Your compassionate response: _____

_____

_____

_____

6. Your harsh thought:_____

_____

_____

_____

Your compassionate response:_____

_____

_____

_____

7. Your harsh thought:_____

_____

_____

_____

Your compassionate response:_____

_____

_____

_____

8. Your harsh thought:_____

_____

_____

_____

Your compassionate response:_____

_____

_____

_____

9. Your harsh thought:_____

_____

_____

_____

Your compassionate response:_____

_____

_____

_____

10. Your harsh thought:_____

_____

_____

_____

Your compassionate response:_____

_____

_____

_____

What Went Wrong?

Do you interpret failure as a signal to stop trying?

You think that because you tried something and it didn't work, that you should just stop. You think failing means something bad and shameful about you.

Lesson 6: Why You Need to Expect to Fail

Today we're going to talk about the dreaded concept of failure.

I'll bet you've thought about failure many times in your weight loss history. Without really thinking about what failure means.

> *Only those who dare to fail greatly can ever achieve greatly.*
>
> ~Robert F. Kennedy

Well, first *let's talk about what it means to you.*

Does it mean not reaching your goal weight?

Having an extra helping of something you honestly weren't hungry for?

Or maybe to you it means that you're beginning another program once again to get rid of some long-term extra pounds.

So you label yourself as a failure.

And most of us tend to think that failure is bad.

But we can look at failure in another way.

Failure is simply feedback. What we tried didn't work. We need to try another method. Another viewpoint. Another strategy.

Failure in weight loss simply means our method wasn't effective. Maybe our thinking needs to be adjusted. Maybe we need a new plan.

But in every "failure," there's a silver lining if we look at it the right way.

Failure can be our key to the perfect path for us to permanent weight loss.

Because looking at what didn't work is a way to eliminate options and focus on what can and will work.

This is one of my favorite concepts, borrowed from the work of John Maxwell in his book *Failing Forward*.

Maxwell's premise is that failure is part of learning. And we should never let it squash our attempts to achieve what we really want. You are definitely going to make mistakes. That is a given. In order to achieve what you want, failure is the price we must pay.

Many of us look at failure differently. We see it as a sign to stop. Something's wrong. Something wrong in particular with us.

In fact, one of my favorite quotes from Failing Forward is,

"If you're not failing, you're probably not really moving forward."

We tend to go along on our path, happy when things are easy and everything is going according to plan. But as soon as we hit a bump in the road, we stop and turn around.

Brooke Castillo, author of *If I Am So Smart, Why Can't I Lose Weight?*, gives a great example of this behavior we've all done and how silly it is when we really take a look at it. Brooke describes how when you go out shopping, you know you are going to encounter some traffic lights. When the lights turn red, you stop, and then when they turn green, you move forward, toward your destination.

Stopping and giving up when we fail at something would be like going shopping, coming to a red light, and turning around and going home.

Oh well, I guess it's not meant to be. Something must be wrong with me. I should just go home.

Imagine!

And yet we treat our weight loss failures as signals to go home. When they're really just red lights.

And when we pause at the red light, all that we should be doing is taking stock. Evaluating.

So we can move ahead with new knowledge and a new perspective.

What happened?

Why did it happen?

What could I have done instead?

Do I know why I chose to do what I did?

If I don't know the answer, where might I look for it?

How can I use this experience of not reaching my goal to help me get there eventually?

Failure can mean something completely different if you are open to it. And I suggest you think of this quote from John Maxwell to help you view things in a whole new light:

"In life, the question is not if you will have problems, but how you are going to deal with your problems. If the possibility of failure were erased, what would you attempt to achieve?"

You can do this.

Change your definition of failure.

Dive deeper into this concept. Go to the corresponding worksheet and do the exercise.

Worksheet 6: Using Your Failure to Move Forward

Anything you've done that you consider a *"failure"* is really an *opportunity* to learn, move forward, and ultimately reach your goal. So I want you to go through this process when you think you've done something that didn't work.

1. What happened? Describe the incident in neutral terms, just the facts.

_____

_____

_____

_____

2. Why did I choose to take these actions? Do not beat yourself up here. Again, just facts.

_____

_____

_____

_____

3. What was I thinking when I did this? And **what was I feeling**?

_____

_____

_____

_____

4. What could I have done instead? What would I have to think to do that new behavior next time?

_____

_____

_____

_____

5. How can I use this error to move forward and grow on my path to weight loss?

_____

_____

_____

_____

What Went Wrong?

Is there a part of you that doesn't want to do what it takes?

Part of you wants to change your habits and do what it takes to lose your extra weight. And yet *there's a part of you that doesn't want to change.* Doesn't want to do the work. And you aren't acknowledging that these two parts of you can co-exist.

Lesson 7: Acknowledge Your Ambivalence

No matter how much you want something, there's always at least a small part of you that wants things to stay just the way they are.

"No way!" I can hear you protest.

"I'm not happy with not feeling or looking my best. I'm ready to do whatever it takes to lose this weight."

But are you?

We all know the most obvious physical and psychological benefits that you stand to gain as your scale number goes down. But unless you acknowledge that you have some natural ambivalence, it may be tough to make any progress toward your weight loss goal.

Let me explain:

Imagine you really want to do something. Your desire is real. You can feel it, taste it, and even smell it as you think about doing this thing. So you set your goal, you get excited, and you begin to take inspired actions.

All is going well.

But sooner or later, you will slow down. You will make a choice that will throw you off track.

And you will run into a brick wall. There goes your goal.

And, then you feel bad. And the beating begins! "Why can't I do this?"

"What's wrong with me?"

There's nothing wrong with you, my friend. You simply forgot to acknowledge your ambivalence. **Ambivalence simply means that you have opposing desires.**

You want two different things. And this creates a conflict.

It's natural to want, more than anything else, to reach your ideal weight range. It's also natural to want to eat whatever you want, whenever you want. In unlimited quantities. Especially if you have unknowingly trained your brain to respond to emotions by turning to food.

What happens then is like a collision.

Two opposing desires run right into each other. And guess which one wins?

The one that you've been practicing more. In this case, eating with abandon wins.

So, if weight loss is your goal, there is definitely something you can do to avoid this collision.

I'm going to walk you through the steps. You can follow

along with the corresponding worksheet. It's called Acknowledging Your Ambivalence.

1. First, let's look at what you'll gain (pardon the pun) by losing weight. What will improve in your life? List things across all life categories, like your appearance, your self-esteem, your relationships, your health, career, or your wardrobe.

2. Now, let's take a look at the benefits of not losing weight. Here's where you'll need to dig a little and be really honest with yourself. For example, if you choose to not lose weight, you can eat whatever you want, whenever you want to, and as much as you want; you can sleep and play instead of exercise, and you never have to say "no" to yourself.

3. Our next step is to take a look at the price you're likely to pay if you don't resolve your weight issue. Things like poor health, not feeling great about yourself, having to dress to hide your weight, or not putting yourself out in the world as much as you might if you felt proud and confident.

4. And finally, let's examine the costs of losing weight, the emotional and physical costs. You might have to evaluate your relationships, to determine if they really support you. Or, say no to food that you're not hungry for, or not eat food that you've decided isn't in your best interest to eat. You might have to find a different way to reward yourself that doesn't involve food. And, learn to give yourself joy in other ways that don't involve eating.

So, fill out this worksheet.

And here's the final step. Acknowledge all the costs of losing weight (how hard it might be), and all the benefits of not losing weight.

Now, take a look at the costs of staying the same and the benefits of losing your extra weight. These two categories are what you will focus on.

At this point, I'd like you to put those lists away.

And use all of your brainpower to stay focused on what will move you forward... the costs of not losing, and the benefits of losing weight.

This is what you should read on a daily or almost daily basis.

And when those pesky thoughts come up about sleeping in when you have an exercise date or are faced with overeating opportunities several times in a week, your brain will have already thought of them. And you will have acknowledged them. But you will have chosen to focus on what you really want: lasting weight loss.

Control what you focus on. You can do this.

Dive deeper into this concept. Go to the corresponding worksheet and do the exercise.

Worksheet 7: Learn to Acknowledge Your Ambivalence

I'm sure you want to end your struggle with weight, food, eating and hating your body. But on some level, *there is always some ambivalence about what we need to do to get the results we want.* Here is a way to make sure you know and face all the hidden costs and benefits of losing weight. Of course you know there are benefits to losing weight. But there are also benefits to staying where you are right now.

Use this worksheet to uncover your mixed feelings, look them in the eye, and then keep your focus where you need it most: on the benefits of losing weight, and the costs of not losing weight.

1. What are the costs of losing weight?

_____

_____

_____

_____

2. What are the benefits of losing weight?

_____

_____

_____

_____

3. What are the costs of not losing weight?

_____

_____

_____

_____

4. What are the benefits of not losing weight?

_____

_____

_____

_____

What Went Wrong?

Are you committed only if it's smooth and easy?

You think you really want to lose weight, but as **soon as you run into a challenging situation, you fade away.** You don't really understand the difference between being committed and being interested.

Lesson 8: Are You Truly Committed? Or Just Interested?

Very often we set a goal, we decide to do it, and then we just stop thinking about it. We're not really clear on what makes some of us reach our goals and others fall down and not get up again.

> *Commitment is an act, not a word.*
>
> ~Jean-Paul Sartre

And sometimes, things come up that cause us to forget that we even set any goals in the first place.

Weight loss is no exception.

What is this problem and how could it impact your own weight loss program?

And how can you avoid it totally and actually reach your goals?

I first heard this concept of "committed or interested" explained by author and coach Linda Spangle in her book *100 Days of Weight Loss*.

Here's the deal:

When we choose and set a goal, we assume that we are committed to it.

But there's a big difference between being committed to a goal and being interested in it. Here's how to tell where you are right now.

When you are committed to your weight loss, you want it with no reservations. You are ready to jump in with both feet, and will do whatever is required of you.

By contrast, when you are merely interested in losing weight, you want it, but with certain conditions. You will follow your program but it depends on what is required of you... in other words, you will follow it if it's easy.

When you are committed to your weight loss, you know you will do what it takes no matter how challenging it might be. You will do what's required no matter what else is happening in your life at this time.

You are truly invested in going the distance.

When you are interested in losing weight, a lot depends on what else you have going on. You have one foot out the door and one foot in your program. In fact, if you are honest with yourself from the beginning, you know that you might not be willing to go the distance.

Committed? It's irrelevant what your mood is when you are following your plan.

Interested? An awful lot hinges on whether your mood is good enough to take action.

When you are truly committed, you make your weight loss an ultimate priority, and you will do whatever it takes to get there.

But when you are interested, although you'd love to reach your goal weight, other things always seem to come first.

Do you recognize yourself here? Which side of the fence are you on: committed? Or interested?

Before you take another step toward weight loss, hit the pause button and ask yourself if you are committed or interested. **If weight loss is really important to you, it's crucial that you jump in with both feet and take some committed actions.**

As you read this if you have a lot of buts, I'd back off and do some self- evaluation. Start your weight loss efforts after you can honestly answer "yes" to all the "committed" questions.

That's how you lose weight.

Dive deeper into this concept. Go to the corresponding worksheet and do the exercise.

Worksheet 8: Learning to Be Committed

In order to make a change in your life, you need to be committed. And many of us assume we are committed when, in fact, we are merely interested.

1. If you are **interested** in doing something, you will stick to your plan when it's convenient, when it's comfortable, and when it's easy. It's not a stretch for you. If something comes up or you become uncomfortable, it's pretty easy to stop working on your plan. List a few examples of some things you are or have been *interested in.*

_____

_____

_____

_____

2. If you are **committed** to doing something, this is a whole different ballgame! You are pushed out of your comfort zone. It's very definitely not comfortable, easy, or convenient. You want it, but it may seem hard. Hard is not bad. *It's not a signal to stop and go home. If you are committed, you can look at "hard" as an invitation to grow as a person.* Please list a few things that you have done in your life that required you to be *committed*, even if it wasn't convenient or easy.

_____

_____

_____

_____

3. Go back to the first question. **When you think about things you were simply interested in, what was your outcome when the road got rough?** What were your results?

_____

_____

_____

_____

4. Now think about the second question. **When you think about things you've done that you were truly committed to, what was your outcome when the road got rough?** What were your results?

_____

_____

_____

_____

What Went Wrong?

Are your expectations realistic?

You have expectations that aren't realistic for you or your body or your lifestyle. So when you don't get results, instead of looking at your expectations, you simply give up while once again assuming it must be you.

Lesson 9: Check Your Expectations

Let's take a look now at **your expectations**.

It's great to have goals. It's great to have goals that are a stretch. But it's disheartening to have goals that are simply not achievable.

Martha Beck, author and life coach, calls goals that are achievable, but are a stretch WIGS. WIGS stands for "wildly improbable goals."

I understand what she means and why she likes to use this to help you pull yourself toward what you want. But I'm not in love with the word "improbable."

If I think something is improbable, that makes it harder for me to try.

So let's just think of your goal and expectation as big, bold and achievable.

If anyone in the world has done what you want to do, then you can find a way to do it.

You want it to be big and bold. There's no point in going for something that's easily within your comfort zone.

We all grow when we push the envelope and work toward something that's feels slightly out of reach.

Now we come to the reality part of our goals.

Is it doable?

It is actually achievable?

Do you want to look like a super model?

Do you really, really want to be 6'1" but you're 5'4"?

Do you want super slim hips but you and your family are created a little wider?

As much as we want to stretch and achieve something that feels like a major accomplishment, we need to make it real.

Something that can actually happen. **To you.**

In your body. In your life.

With your genetics. And with your level of commitment.

That still leaves plenty of room for big and bold.

We're just adding a dose of reality. And making these goals achievable.

So read what you have written so far about your goal (not just the number on the scale) and give it the reality test... Is it doable?

If so, go on to the next lesson.

If not, let's go back and tweak it until it is real and possible for you.

Dive deeper into this concept. Go to the corresponding worksheet and do the exercise.

Worksheet 9: Create Great Expectations

If you're in the habit of setting goals like losing extra weight and consistently don't reach these goals, it's time to take a look at your expectations.

Goals give you a chance to dream and aim for the stars, but if you're not in the right galaxy, you won't get where you want to go.

Here's how it works:

1. Your goal: to be fit and healthy (this is an example.... fill in your own answer.)

_____

_____

_____

_____

2. Has anyone achieved this goal? Who are they?

_____

_____

_____

_____

3. Do you know what you need to do to get there?
What are your next action steps? What is your big picture
plan?

_____

_____

_____

_____

4. Are there any skills you need to learn? If there are,
how can you get the knowledge you need?

_____

_____

_____

_____

5. Is this goal possible within your life and your body?

_____

_____

_____

_____

6. Do you need support?

_____

_____

_____

_____

7. Are you willing to do what it takes?

_____

_____

_____

_____

If you can answer these questions and are willing to do what it takes, congratulations! Your expectations are real and achievable.

If not, go back to the drawing board. How can you adapt your goal to fit the rest of the criteria... and make it doable by you?

What Went Wrong?

Do you compare yourself to everyone around you?

You are constantly comparing yourself to everyone around you. You want to be able to eat what your friend eats, weigh what a movie star weighs, and have the willpower of a saint. **Your comparisons will do nothing but keep you stuck.**

Lesson 10: Don't Compare and Despair

Often when we want to achieve something, instead of looking inside ourselves and seeing what would be right for us, what would make us feel great and what would be a cool personal stretch, we look around.

We look outside ourselves.

Just to see what everyone else is doing.

How much they weigh. How they dress. How attractive they are. Their money. Their husband. And their home.

It can be an endless comparison.

It takes up a lot of time and mental energy.

And here's the funny thing: **what others are doing has nothing to do with us and what *we're* trying to achieve.**

When we look inside ourselves and get to know what matters to us (a pretty unique concoction), we are able to innovate and create.

When we look to others to see what they are doing, something that's hard to not do on Facebook, we tend to shrink.

That's because when we compare, we usually are likely to despair. (This is an old saying.)

Your goal is not to be as good as someone else, as thin or as pretty as someone else, or as happy as someone else.

Your goal is to aim for the best version of yourself that you can create.

In order to do this, you must put some blinders on.

Stop comparing.

You might notice what others are doing.

But stay in your own space.

Compare and despair keeps you stuck. Because there will always be someone better than you at something.

But to innovate and create, you've got all you need.

You, your imagination, and your unique blend of talent.

When you are creating your weight loss vision, focus only on you.

Dive deeper into this concept. Go to the corresponding worksheet and do the exercises.

Worksheet 10: Escape from Comparing and Despairing

Are you in the habit of comparing yourself to everyone on your radar? It doesn't work, does it? It doesn't motivate you; in fact it can actually be demotivating.

We are all individuals and our goal is simply to be the best we can be. Not to be as good as your friends on Facebook, just to be your personal best. Yet *it's hard to see how other women eat, or look, or dress, and not measure ourselves by their yardstick.*

Instead of comparing, which usually leads to despairing, let's take a different tactic. **Look at people you admire. Notice the qualities they have... the way they eat, the way they move their bodies in exercise, and the way they take care of themselves. And then ask yourself: how can I learn from her? And most importantly, how does she think to get the results she has?**

Remember to look at traits that are *possible* for you. Or think about what you are envying and imagine some version of that for yourself.

If you do compare and don't want to despair, ask yourself:

1. What is it I wish I had / could do?

_____

_____

_____

_____

2. Is this possible for me?

_____

_____

_____

_____

3. What did she do to achieve that?

_____

_____

_____

_____

4. What did she think to get herself to take those actions?

_____

_____

_____

_____

5. Am I willing to do what it takes?

_____

_____

_____

_____

6. Can I talk to her and ask her about her perspective and learn how she did it?

_____

_____

_____

_____

What Went Wrong?

Do you think getting what you want should be easy?

When you are trying to reach a goal and it is difficult for you, you assume that anything that is hard is too hard, and you stop trying. You also think that when something is hard, that it's not fair. You think things should be easier for you.

Lesson 11: Learn Why "Hard" Is Good and How to Stop Thinking "Easy" Is Your Goal

How often have you heard yourself say, "But it's so hard!" I can certainly think of more than a few times that phrase has come out of my mouth.

When you say something is hard, how do you feel?

I know I feel burdened, overwhelmed, and a little hopeless with a touch of dread. Who would want to put effort into something that feels unpleasant right from the beginning?

When we think something is hard, our knee-jerk reaction is to feel bad, and then either avoid it like the plague or go into it grudgingly, waiting for the sky to fall.

When we feel dread, hopelessness, or a sense of being overwhelmed, we tend to give very little effort (why bother?) or do it kind of half-assed because we think we'll probably fail anyway (because it's so hard).

Not a great way to start. Weight loss. Or any project in your life.

Wouldn't it be cool to start approaching a goal with excitement, zest, or, at least, peace?

You can. Here's how.

We need to reframe the idea of "hard." And think about why it's come to mean something negative.

What types of things do we usually label as hard?

> -Things that take us outside of our comfort zone,
>
> -things that make us stretch beyond what we expected or what was required, and
>
> -things that have no immediate payoff... no instant gratification. (You mean I have to eat mindfully and stay connected to myself and exercise *without* seeing an immediate ten-pound weight loss?)

But here's a new way to look at the concept of hard. Who says hard has to be something bad? Or something to be avoided at all costs?

We are wired to actually like hard things. Humans are given the intellectual ability to figure things out. Problems stimulate us. If we approach them the right way.

For example, we know that if you think, "That's hard," you might feel dread.

If you think, instead, "Wow, that's challenging," you might feel stimulated and even excited.

Sometimes, we tend to think that we want life to be easy peasy. No problems, no hurdles, no learning curve, just simple.

Well, guess what? It's not really true. Well, of course we don't want mountains to climb over everything we do in life. We'd all love things to go smoothly. But when they don't, remember that **our brains are designed to find solutions to everything we encounter. We can find solutions.**

Just imagine how differently you might go through life if your motto was "I can figure this out," instead of "Oh, no! A problem!"

When you are beginning a new weight loss program, check the conversation that's going on in your mind. If you find yourself worrying about how hard it's going to be, you are setting yourself up to start your program with a big weight on your shoulders. Not exactly a fun way to live and get things done.

But, if you can think about starting a new weight loss program and accept that *there will be challenges*, you'll feel differently, and will be so much more likely to look for solutions and do well!

Be interested and compassionate as you tune into your own mind.

Take a few minutes to go back in time to the last couple of weight loss efforts you made. Did you go into those programs thinking about how hard it was going to be?

Now, it's time for a fresh start.

By seeing roadblocks as temporary challenges that you can figure out, you are MUCH more likely to stick to your program, reach your goals, and feel great while doing so.

If you can begin to catch yourself when you start thinking things shouldn't be so darn hard, you will benefit from changing your mantra to "I've got this!"

Take a moment to explore how you usually react to challenges and see how easy it is to create new responses to life's little, or big, trials.

Dive deeper into this concept. Go to the corresponding worksheet and do the exercise.

Worksheet 11: Learn to Welcome Doing "Hard" Things

If you're past the age of twelve, you've probably figured out that life can be challenging. And if we fear and shy away from challenges, we don't grow. If we fear hard things, we can never get what we really want, unless our desires are small and easy. And when we do go through challenging times and come out the other side, we are stronger. We feel great! Our image of our self expands and we feel like we can take on the world.

Your goal is to stop being put off by hard things. View them instead as things that are valuable and worth striving for. Weight loss doesn't have to be a struggle, yet it may not be simple, either.

Let's take a look at your current attitude toward hard things.

1. Think of a time you went through a big challenging experience. After you got through it, think about how you felt.

_____

_____

_____

_____

2. In that situation, what did you tell yourself when you ran into roadblocks? Did it feel good or bad?

_____

_____

_____

_____

3. What is your general inner motto? Is it more often "Oh, no!!!" or is it "I'll figure it out?"

_____

_____

_____

_____

**4. When you say, "Oh no, this is going to be hard,"
what feelings come up for you?**

_____

_____

_____

_____

**5. What actions do these feelings make you want to
take?**

_____

_____

_____

_____

**6. When you say "I'll figure it out," what feelings
come up for you?**

_____

_____

_____

_____

7. What actions do these feelings make you want to take?

_____

_____

_____

_____

8. Which path makes sense for you going forward?

_____

_____

_____

_____

9. Can you think of someone in your life to use as a model who deals with life's challenges in a positive way?

_____

_____

_____

_____

10. Are you willing to notice how you respond to challenges and begin to move just one degree in the opposite direction? (Assuming you aren't already thinking "I've got this!")

_____

_____

_____

_____

What Went Wrong?

Do you hate yourself at your current weight?

You hate yourself, your body, and your weight. *You can't find anything to be happy about until you reach a certain number.* This leaves you feeling awful right now and makes moving forward extremely difficult.

Lesson 12: What's Perfect about Where You Are Today?

Yes, I do know that you are now questioning my sanity.

How could things be perfect at your current weight?

Do I know how you feel in a bathing suit?

Have you even tried on a bathing suit in the last ten years?

In the process of clearing our path for permanent weight loss, we not only need to look at what patterns caused us to fail in the past, but **we need to make peace with where we are right now.**

Now, I can hear you loud and clear. The first thing I do with my clients is have a Let's Get Started session where we do what you are doing in this series of lessons; we look at what worked, what didn't work, and make a plan to move forward.

Most clients don't want to do this.

They want to get down to business yesterday.

"Just tell me what to eat! I don't want to waste time thinking about my past diets. And of course I hate my body and weight now! Who wouldn't?"

These are some of the things they think about themselves when we first meet:

> *"This weight is terrible!"*

> *"I absolutely can't be happy until I lose twenty-seven pounds."*

> *"I hate myself for not being able to lose this weight and keep it off!"*

That's an awful lot of negative energy to carry around, don't you think?

That negative energy is heavy. It takes up valuable real estate in your beautiful mind that could be spent moving you forward and getting you where you want to go.

So we can't approach change from a place of hatred. It simply makes change a zillion times harder.

Hatred for yourself, your body, your life.

Change that comes from peace, love, and acceptance flows much more easily and feels amazing.

How do we get to this place of self-acceptance right now?

And be able to see ourselves at our current weight as "perfect?"

We focus on the good.

We look for the lessons we've learned by reaching this moment, in this body, at this weight.

Right now, we are perfect.

If we hadn't gained this weight, and been through all the drama we've been through, and wound up right here, we never would find ourselves on the verge of a massive life shift.

You know the old saying that if you keep doing what you've always done, you'll get what you've always gotten?

Well, that is exactly true.

Right now your weight is perfect. It is a reminder that you need to reconnect to yourself and give yourself what you really need.

Hint: the Snickers Ice Cream bar is not what you really need... that's a poor substitute.

So where do you begin to be able to see your present life and your weight as perfect?

First, stop arguing with reality. Right now, you weigh X. That is your truth. When you can take a deep breath and own it, then you can move forward.

You are this weight because you took care of yourself in the only way you knew. Looking back, you can clearly see that the choices you made didn't give you the results you really wanted.

But that is what you did. And now you have your results.

Byron Katie, creator of The Work, a brilliant method of

looking at your thoughts and your life, likes to say: *When you argue with reality you will lose... but only 100% of the time.*

Second, know that by focusing on the positive perspective of why you weigh X, you will feel better. You'll breathe a sign of peace and relief.

And from that place of feeling better, you will take actions that will bring you closer to the amazing results you want.

So, what's perfect about your weight right now?

Dive deeper into this concept. Go to the corresponding worksheet and do the exercise.

Worksheet 12: Appreciating Where You Are Today

────────────────────────

It's really imperative that you be happy now, at your current weight, before you can move forward. Or at least kind and compassionate toward yourself no matter what your scale says.

When I ask *what's perfect about where you are today, many clients find it impossible to even consider that there's anything at all good about where they are right now.*

But everything you've done, all the choices you've made, brought you to this place. *And although we tend to be unhappy about some aspect of our present moment, it's never true that all that led to this point was "bad."*

So what I'd like you to do is take a look at yourself right now, whatever you weigh. *See if you can shift your perspective ever so slightly to allow yourself to see the good, even if you're not where you want to be yet.*

Right now, **I weigh**:

1. This extra weight is mostly the result of:

_____

_____

_____

_____

2. If it wasn't for this extra weight, I would never have realized that I am:

_____

_____

_____

_____

3. If it wasn't for this extra weight, I might not have gotten in touch with my:

_____

_____

_____

_____

4. Because of this weight, I now know I need to give myself:

_____

_____

_____

_____

5. This weight has gotten my attention, and now I know that I need to honor my:

_____

_____

_____

_____

6. My weight has forced me to slow down and really take a look at:

_____

_____

_____

_____

7. The process of focusing on my body and my eating has put me in touch with my:

_____

_____

_____

_____

8. If it wasn't for this extra weight, I might have missed out on:

_____

_____

_____

_____

What Went Wrong?

Can you truly visualize being at your goal weight?

You know what you want to weigh, but you don't really have a vision. You think things will change for you at a certain weight but you're not sure why or how.

Lesson 13: What Do You Really, Really Want?

What do you want?

When we don't have a very clear picture of what we want, it should come as no surprise that it's rare to get it.

Yet we are. Surprised. Constantly.

We're surprised when our body doesn't change and yet we have no clear idea of what we want our end result to look like.

Well, in order to get the result you want in the realm of weight loss or anything else, you first have to give your brain a clear version of what you're going after.

When your brain gets this message, and it's reinforced often, your mind will come up with supportive thoughts. Voila!

Those supportive thoughts will give you strong, positive feelings.

And those strong, positive feelings will help you take the actions required to give you those results you crave.

A lovely circle of think—feel—act, and then you get your result.

So if weight loss is what you want, it's crucial to go deep into your desire. Let's play a game called **The Miracle Question**.

If you look at the worksheet with this lesson, you can follow along. This will give you your own personal blueprint of what you want.

The value of this?

Priceless, when you are looking for motivation to keep on keeping on.

This is how you create the drive that will pull you forward toward your weight loss goal.

Read along with me and then go to the worksheet from this lesson and fill in your own answers to the Miracle Question.

Here's how it goes:

Imagine that you have a problem. (You do. You want to lose weight and you haven't been successful so far.)

Play with me here.

You go to bed and sleep peacefully through the night.

When you awake, wonder of wonders, you are now in

your body, in your real life, but without the extra weight.

Gone! Poof!

What does that look like?

What does it feel like?

Walk around. How does your body feel? Can you move differently?

What do you notice about sitting and standing and walking without the extra weight?

Now get dressed. Are you choosing something to wear that you never were able to wear before? How do you look? Take a good look in the mirror. Do you like what you see? Why?

Go about your day.

How do people treat you in this new version of your body?

Do you act differently? How do you relate to your friends? Your family? Your coworkers?

Picture yourself walking down the street, going into shops, dealing with strangers. Is there a difference in how you feel, act and carry yourself?

I want you to spend some time fleshing this vision out.

Imagine that this little mental video is a preview of your future life.

Make it in color with details. And read it often.

It's so much easier to be pulled toward something that is irresistible, than to push yourself toward something that feels like hard work.

Dive deeper into this concept. Go to the corresponding worksheet and do the exercise.

Worksheet 13: The Miracle Question

When you are trying to envision a future without binge eating or emotional eating and the extra weight they bring, it can be hard to see past your situation right now.

Back in the 1980's, therapists Steven de Shazer and Insoo Kim Berg developed a branch of psychology called Solution Focused Brief Therapy. One of their most widely used tools that allowed clients to envision what they wanted is this: **The Miracle Question**. Follow along and fill in the blanks, and you will get a detailed picture of what you are working toward.

Imagine that you go to bed tonight. And while you are sleeping, a miracle occurs. The eating problem and the extra weight that you struggle with are gone. *You are at your natural weight.*

1. You wake up and get out of bed, washing up and getting dressed. How are things different? What's it like looking in the mirror? How do you move? Feel? What does your body look like?

_____

_____

_____

_____

2. You move through your day. What happens when you sit down and eat breakfast? How are things at work? What is your demeanor like? How do people respond to you? What's different?

_____

_____

_____

_____

3. What happens when you go to lunch? Are you acting differently? How about when you choose what to order in a restaurant?

_____

_____

_____

_____

4. You leave work and stop at the grocery store before coming home to cook dinner... What's different for you being in the store? How are you thinking about dinner? What are you cooking?

_____

_____

_____

_____

5. It's the end of your day. Are you feeling a different level of energy than you usually feel? What are your plans for dinner? For the evening? How is this different than what is typical for you?

_____

_____

_____

_____

6. Looking at your day, overall, what feels the same and what feels different if this miracle had occurred and your weight was no longer an issue?

_____

_____

_____

_____

7. If zero (0) represented the worst feeling, and the best feeling was rated at a 10, what number were you after the miracle occurred? And in your real life, what number are you at now? What would have to happen to move you up the number scale one notch higher, right now?

_____

_____

_____

_____

What Went Wrong?

Why do you want to lose weight?

You have a goal, but you aren't clear on why you want it. *You are focused only on the superficial reasons for wanting to be a certain number or certain size.*

Lesson 14: Why Do You Want It?

Your next question is: Why do you want it? I mean, *really*.

Why is losing weight important to you?

Maybe your answer is so that you can look better.

Now go deeper. Why do you want to look better?

Maybe your answer is to be your best version of yourself? Or to have more energy? Or to overcome a health issue related to your weight.

> *To be fully engaged in our lives, we must have bigger and bolder goals.*
>
> *Why do you do what you do?*
>
> *Do you really know?*
>
> *Do the people around you know?*
>
> ~Jason M. Womack

All good reasons. But I want you to go underneath these reasons.

And figure out WHY you really want this.

If the Miracle Question gives you a map that shows you exactly where you are going, the Why question will give you gas in your car to help you get there. It will give you extra motivation that is like jet fuel for your desire.

So, let's take a look at your why.

Whenever we want something, whether it's a good mate, a great job, money, or a fit body, we don't just want what that will bring to us physically.

What we really want is how we believe it will make us feel when we get it.

So when you look at your surface reason, which is very valid, it's really the way it will make you feel that will give you motivation.

If you want to be healthy, maybe you want that so you can feel vibrant, alive, and proud.

If you want to look great and be able to comfortably wear a bathing suit at the beach, maybe you want that so you can feel confident, excited, and gratified.

And if you want to earn a certain amount of money, maybe you want to do that so you can feel secure and competent.

The bottom line is, we all want different things in our lives.

Partly, we want these things because of what they can do for us, and what we can do with them. *But mainly,*

we want them for the feelings we give ourselves when we have them.

So we are always going after a feeling.

Later on in this book, I will show you how you can create some of those feelings now.

Right now, before you have even lost one pound.

But for now, dig deep to understand and articulate why you want to lose weight. And how you think it will make you feel.

Say it out loud. Acknowledge it to yourself. You are going for the weight loss. **And** the feeling you believe you will get when you have it.

Dive deeper into this concept. Go to the corresponding worksheet and do the exercise.

Worksheet 14: Discovering Why You Want It

Now that the Miracle Question has helped you paint your detailed picture of what you are working toward, *let's go deeper and figure out WHY you want to lose weight and conquer your eating issues.*

Just about everything we want is driven by our desire to *feel* a certain way... We think it's about reaching a certain number on the scale, or a certain size jeans, or even finally wearing a bathing suit.

But it's all about how those things will make you feel.

So dig in and take a look at what feeling you are going after.

Repeat this process for every reason you uncover. When you are finished, I want you to look at your life and ask yourself: **How can I begin to create the feelings I want right now, before I reach my goal?**

1. Why do you want to lose weight?

_____

_____

_____

_____

2. What will you feel if you accomplish this?

_____

_____

_____

_____

3. Go deeper... Why is it important to feel_____?

_____

_____

_____

_____

4. I want to_____so I can_____so I can feel_____.

_____

_____

_____

_____

5. Right now, to feel_____, I can begin to think or do_____.

_____

_____

_____

_____

What Went Wrong?

How do you motivate yourself?

You look outside yourself for motivation. You believe that a certain person or activity will keep you pumped up and motivated, and you don't realize that motivation is an inside job. Once you lose your motivation, you have no idea how to get it back.

Lesson 15: You Need to Be Able to Create Your Own Motivation

Lots of women sign up to work with me because they hear I'm a great motivator. But actually, this isn't true.

No one can motivate you to lose weight.

Motivation is something you create. It comes from deep inside you and that's good news. Because you can bring it up any time you need it.

Motivation is the internal process for creating the desire and energy that guide you toward something you want. It's an inside job. That's why *although we can get support from others, we can't really ask them to motivate us.*

To start creating your own motivation, pick a real, achievable goal. One that you can visualize yourself reaching. If it's too big or not realistic, it can actually be de-motivating! If the goal itself makes you feel great thinking about it, that alone will help you create your motivation.

Make some time every day to think of your end game... and in particular not just what you will achieve, or how much you will weigh, or what kinds of clothing you'll be able to wear, but focus more on how you will feel.

Keep motivating yourself until you create a habit of focusing on what you want to get yourself to move forward.

And find a balance between focusing on how far you've come, and how far you have yet to go.

For example, let's say you want to lose fifty pounds total, and you've just lost ten. *Do* be excited about the ten you've lost, and do allow yourself to do a happy dance around your house.

But also keep in mind that there are forty more pounds to go. If you only focus on the ten you've lost, you might celebrate those ten pounds right back on your body. And if you only focus on the forty more pounds left to lose, you might begin to feel hopeless and think that this is too much work.

Keep alternating back and forth to motivate yourself to keep going. It's a little like a seesaw that keeps you moving up and down and aiming for that middle balance.

Give yourself some rewards for what you've accomplished. And let those accomplishments to date give you fuel to keep you fired up about continuing. After all, if you've lost even one pound, all you have to do is repeat what you've done forty-nine more times.

Know there will be lulls and setbacks. But you can always

reach inside and pull out your own motivation any day of the week.

You are in charge of keeping your internal desire up so that you keep moving forward.

You fall down, you get back up. Of course you can do this!

Dive deeper into this concept. Go to the corresponding worksheet and do the exercise.

Worksheet 15: Creating Your Own Motivation

Even if you were one of my private clients, creating your own motivation is something you'd have to do for yourself. Your friends, family, or coach can be your support, but motivation is an inside job. Every day you need to find a way to keep moving ahead toward your weight loss goals. And creating motivation is a sure way to keep you moving ahead.

On a regular basis, you need to review what you want. Why you want it. How achieving it will make you feel. These things will fuel your desire even when challenges appear in your path.

Here are some examples of how you can create motivation for yourself:

1. *Review your vision (written) of what you are hoping to achieve.*

2. *Take a look at your big WHY. Why do you want to lose weight?*

3. *Pause and really imagine how you will feel when you lose your weight and it is no longer an issue in your life.*

4. *Write about your feelings in a journal, so you can feel them and not stuff them down with Oreos.*

5. *Meditate... slow your brain down and listen to your breathing.*

6. *Give yourself a meaningful reward for what you've accomplished so far.*

7. *Think of another meaningful reward to give yourself when you reach the goal that's still ahead.*

8. *Connect with a friend and talk about any challenges you are having.*

Ok, now it's your turn.

This is your job... What can YOU do to create motivation that will pull you forward toward your goal? Think about things to do in the morning, midday, and at the end of your day as needed.

Morning:

1.

2.

3.

4.

Midday:

1.

2.

3.

4.

Evening:

1.

2.

3.

4.

Think of routines you can do alone, and what you can do with a support person.

What Went Wrong?

Do you know exactly what kinds of errors you made?

You don't think about what types of errors you made in your past efforts to lose weight. You lump it all into one big failure category, with you as the main creator. You are immobilized.

Lesson 16: Begin to Understand Your Errors in Past Weight Loss Efforts

---

Now it's time to look at your past weight loss efforts and begin to evaluate what went wrong.

Were you not motivated to get a strong start?

> *Do not be embarrassed by your failures. Learn from them and start over.*
>
> ~Richard Branson

You need a strong vision of why you are losing weight and how you want things to look for you.

Did you get a strong start but eventually hit the wall when your momentum petered out?

It's imperative that you learn how to keep yourself on track and get up when you fall down.

Did you have a slow start with your weight loss and allow impatience to throw you off track?

Part of a big goal like weight loss involves knowing you're in this for the long haul... It takes consistent action over long periods of time.

Do you want a really quick fix? Then be prepared to get a short-lived solution.

Or maybe you actually lost your extra weight, and then struggled to keep it off.

How about your emotions? Were you an emotional eater? Did you use food to feel better?

And how about cravings? Are you a binge-eater? At the mercy of frequent cravings for your favorite sweet or starchy carb?

Begin to classify your past errors... What went wrong?

Be curious and play detective.

Your answers to the questions you just read will give you valuable information that will guide your next effort and make you more successful than you've ever been.

Why?

Because you are doing a rewind.

Turning back the story to the beginning and seeing where the heroine started to slide down the slippery slope.

Ok, she did slide down. It's done.

But you will use that knowledge of what you did wrong to give you a much better result this time around.

Beating yourself up is not only not required, but consider it prohibited.

The idea is to use all the clues you can gather from your past weight loss efforts and transform those errors into a road map of exactly where all your potholes are.

When we know our patterns, we can plan for them and make a detour.

Just because you fell into the pothole last time doesn't mean you will this time.

The very fact that you are reading this lesson and clearing your path will help you be guided to be your best self as you lose the extra weight you've accumulated.

Also, consider that while you may have made some errors in the actions you took, nothing really went wrong.

You are here right now.

All those errors and choices have brought you to this perfect time and place to lose your weight once and for all.

Doesn't it feel good to know that by looking at what went wrong, you are increasing the odds for you to do what's needed this time?

Dive deeper into this concept. Go to the corresponding worksheet and do the exercise.

Worksheet 16: Figure Out What Went Wrong

It's not you. I mean, there is nothing wrong with you.

But if you haven't been able to stop overeating or bingeing or eating emotionally, then you have been doing some things that need to change. It's not personal. It's your behavior.

So the purpose of this exercise is to *play detective and begin to classify what areas you need to work on in order to lose weight.*

When you start a weight loss program again, *use this information as a guide. It will tell you exactly where you have a learning opportunity.*

1. Did you understand how to create your own motivation that you could draw on when needed?

_____

_____

_____

_____

2. Did you create a strong vision of what you wanted and why you wanted it?

_____

_____

_____

_____

3. Did you have a plan to pull yourself up for the times you'd inevitably fall down?

_____

_____

_____

_____

4. Were your expectations realistic for your life and your body?

_____

_____

_____

_____

5. Did you learn to manage your emotions so you didn't use food to change the way you felt?

_____

_____

_____

_____

6. Did you restrict what you ate so that you felt deprived?

_____

_____

_____

_____

7. When you made an error, did you mentally beat yourself up, making yourself feel awful?

_____

_____

_____

_____

8. Did you allow food to be your only joy?

_____

_____

_____

_____

9. Did you neglect to take care of yourself, physically, emotionally, or spiritually?

_____

_____

_____

_____

10. Did you focus on what went well or what went wrong?

_____

_____

_____

_____

11. Did you ask for help or support when you needed it?

_____

_____

_____

_____

Now, the purpose of this exercise is NOT to beat yourself again for what you did or didn't do. It's to open your eyes to all the different ways you could now upgrade your efforts next time.

We can't go back in time.

But we can absolutely learn from our past actions.

What Went Wrong?

Are you aware of your patterns and themes?

You think there were random things here and there that didn't work. You don't realize that there are patterns and themes that were created by you. And *if you can see these patterns, you can find a way out of them.*

Lesson 17: What Patterns Are Emerging for You?

Whether you realize it or not, you have many patterns in your life. **Patterns are the habitual ways we think, feel, and act over and over again.** *You may have a pattern of thinking that you did something wrong.*

Or thinking that others know better than you.

Or that you never have enough. (My old personal favorite.)

These are thought patterns.

Our brain is wired to let us repeat things that we do over and over again very efficiently.

So if we get the slightest inkling that it's not fair that others are eating and we aren't, our brain will get right on the job of creating the pattern of "there's never enough."

The thoughts we have on a regular basis help create our lives.

When we think something over and over again, it becomes a habit or a pattern that we don't question. It just is. Eventually, these thought patterns give us our reality.

You may have some patterns of feeling a certain way.

When you are alone, you may be in a pattern of feeling lonely.

So if someone cancels plans with you, you probably go right into your pattern of feeling lonely.

And when you fall off the wagon from the eating path you were on, you may go right into the pattern of feeling hopeless and believing something is wrong with you.

Of course you know that you can also have patterns of behavior... how you act. A perfect example of a pattern of thought *and* behavior is when we tell ourselves, "I can't eat just one" and when we have one potato chip, we continue on to finish the bag.

The good news is that our brains created all of our patterns as a way of making our lives easier and more efficient.

Our brains don't really think or know the consequences of the patterns they help us create. They are simply like an alarm clock we have set to go off at a certain time.

And they will keep doing it, whether it's helpful or not.

To change your patterns, which you will need to do to get a different result, you will first have to become aware of what your patterns are.

Take a look at the worksheet for this day's lesson. Begin

by thinking of things you have done on your quest for weight loss.

What are your habitual thoughts that lead you to overeat? What feelings usually have you reaching for Doritos?

And what actions do you take on a regular basis that keep you from ever reaching your goals?

Since you created your patterns, be assured you can change them. And the first step is really exploring what these patterns are.

Start with your worksheet.

Bringing these patterns to light will ensure they won't be controlling you and sabotaging your weight loss efforts anymore. You are in charge!

Dive deeper into this concept. Go to the corresponding worksheet and do the exercise.

Worksheet 17: Discovering Your Patterns

If you consider yourself a weight loss dropout, you probably stand under an umbrella of failure. What I mean is that because you still want to lose some extra weight, you think that everything you did didn't work. That you did everything wrong. But the reality is that you probably did some things well, and did some things that you may want to change or eliminate. It isn't really helpful to lump everything together and just assume you can't do it... that you can't do anything right. Because that just isn't true.

So it's time to stop putting everything together and going all black and white. Let's separate the fact from the fiction. **Some things you did well. Some things you did and need to do more of. Some things you might want to do less of. And it's a mixture. Your own secret formula for weight loss success.**

Let's think back over the last few years in all your cumulative weight loss efforts.

1. What were you able to do that was helpful?

_____

_____

_____

_____

2. What did you do a little of that you know you could do more of?

_____

_____

_____

_____

3. What did you do that you'd love to stop doing?

_____

_____

_____

_____

4. What did you do that you'd like to do less of?

_____

_____

_____

_____

Now you have a recipe personalized for you. It might look something like this example I made up from a mixture of my clients:

> "I was really good at planning my week and making sure I had good things to eat that were ready and available. I was good at bringing delicious lunches to work and making dates to work out with friends.
>
> I'd like to be more adventurous and cook and prepare some different foods. I tend to get bored with what I cooked and ate each week. I'd also like to make more time for myself: to think, to read, to write, and to just reflect about my life.
>
> I'd love to stop reaching for sweets and starches when I'm upset. I know food isn't the answer to dealing with my emotions, and I'm not sure what is. But I'd love to find out what will really make me feel better when I'm worried or stressed.

I want to do less zoning out... When I'm with others who are eating, I tend to automatically join in whether I'm hungry or not. It's like I forget I'm even trying to lose weight. And I'd like to do less feeling sorry for myself. I know that when I start thinking I'm deprived, I start craving comfort foods and rebelliously start eating."

So there you go. By answering these questions like the example above, you are plotting your new roadmap, using your own patterns from past weight loss efforts.

What Went Wrong?

Is perfect your only standard?

You expect things to work perfectly. You expect yourself to take perfect actions and get perfect results. And when this doesn't happen, you simply give up.

Lesson 18: Leave Perfectionism at the Doorstep

Do you think that in order to lose weight you need to do everything perfectly? And if you don't, then you need to start over? Or maybe just give up?

Perfectionism is the enemy of achieving any goal.

Think about your previous efforts to lose weight. As soon as you slip and do something that isn't serving you, you go back to the starting line to begin over again. And again. And again.

It's really hard to make progress this way, right?

As human beings, none of us are perfect in any way. And yet when trying to lose weight, we expect ourselves to do it without error... no faltering and never a wrong choice.

Reality is that along the path to permanent weight loss, you are slated to make mistakes (remember Lesson 6, Why you need to expect to fail).

Yet too many of us try to beat ourselves into perfection

only to be halted at the starting gate... because we can never be perfect enough.

Does this sound familiar?

> -You experience extreme frustration if you make a mistake.
>
> -You tend to give up quickly if you don't make perfect progress.
>
> -You focus on what you've done wrong instead of what you've done right.
>
> -Or, you spend a lot of time obsessing over small details, to insure that you do things "correctly" and ignore the bigger picture of what you are trying to do.

All of these traits point to perfectionism. And perfectionism simply won't get you where you want to go. Think of it as the adversary of taking action.

What you can do is make an effort to be mindful of when your perfectionism starts rearing its head. As soon as you hear a critical voice in your head telling you that you didn't do something well enough, wake up.

Accept that as a human being you will not do things perfectly. And that's okay.

In fact, it helps to look at your flaws and see what you can love about them.

Look at the big picture of life and ask yourself if what isn't perfect even matters in the long view of things... and if it really doesn't, don't waste another moment beating yourself... just move on.

Your goal is to aim for progress, not perfection.

Progress implies growth and movement.

Perfection implies precision and flawlessness that is simply not a trait that most of us possess.

Stop looking for it!

Dive deeper into this concept. Go to the corresponding worksheet and do the exercise.

Worksheet 18: How to Leave Perfectionism at the Doorstep

Your goal is to begin to take actions and aim for a B instead of an A+.

This is not to say that you shouldn't do your best in any endeavor. But if you fall short, *it's really important not to negate the progress you've already made. And when you let perfectionism be your guide that is exactly what happens. You take actions that aren't perfect, so you give up and add to the damage and then beat yourself up.*

Don't stop.

Just see where you are. Keep going.

And know that sometimes your life grade might be a B. And that's okay.

Exercise: Imagine this: you plan what you're going to eat for the day, but a friend surprises you and brings over a bag full of your favorite candy. You indulge and eat some of it.

A. Old way—You eat it and say, "What the heck, I've blown it!" finish all the candy plus more, and overeat until you go to bed... ready to start over tomorrow.

B. New way—You see where you are and make a mental note without judgment of what you did and your thoughts leading up to it.

C. You let go—You let go of this eating incident and stay on your path for the rest of the day.

D. You continue—You continue on track with a small bump in the road instead of a complete roadblock. No starting over. No self-beating. No saying "What the heck!"

Now it's your turn:

Imagine that you are on your path, living your life and trying to stop eating without hunger. But something happens to derail you. Let's walk through the process of planning out some possible ways you might handle this using the model above:

1. What would you have done in the past? (Your old way of dealing with this.)

_____

_____

_____

_____

2. Where are you now? Evaluate.

_____

_____

_____

_____

3. How can you let go and move on while staying on your path?

_____

_____

_____

_____

4. How will you continue for the rest of the day?

_____

_____

_____

_____

What Went Wrong?

Do you know what stops you from reaching your goals?

You have clear goals. But you keep bumping into the same roadblocks. You have no idea why this keeps happening to you. *You're not aware of the beliefs you hold under the surface that create your successes and failures.*

Lesson 19: Do Your Goals (Secretly) Conflict with Your Beliefs?

Have you ever really, really wanted something? And did everything you thought you could to get it? But never really got what you wanted?

This happens quite a bit with weight loss goals.

We have a goal in mind... to stop eating so much junk food, to start eating only when you're really hungry, or maybe it's to move your body more.

And despite our plans, we just never achieve our goals.

We can't figure out what the problem is, and we begin to think that there's something major wrong with us.

It almost feels like you're sabotaging yourself! And why would you do that?

The thing is **we all have many different beliefs. These beliefs, whether we are aware of them or not, actually shape our lives. And, they determine whether or not we reach our goals.**

Here's what I mean:

-Your goal is to lose weight. You think you want this with all your heart, and yet you keep stopping at the McDonalds' drive through on the way home... You eat a big Mac **and** your dinner. Why? Because you have a secret belief that it's simply not fair that other people can eat fast food and you have to say no to yourself.

-Maybe your goal is to get a promotion at work, and for this to happen, you need to complete a big project. *You keep putting it* on your calendar and yet you never get around to working on it. Why? Because your hidden belief is that life shouldn't be hard. And this project feels hard.

-Or, maybe your goal is to be healthier by exercising and to get a good report from your family doctor. So why does it feel impossible to get yourself to the gym? I'll bet your underlying belief is that life is short, and it's no fun to work out when you could be watching television.

So these secret or not-so-secret beliefs that we hold cause us to feel a certain way and then take certain actions.

If we believe life is short and should be all play and no work, then no amount of rewards or bargaining are going to get you to the gym.

What can we do about this so we can set goals and not stand in our own way?

1. First, when you keep setting a goal and keep thwarting your own success, *zero in on the belief that's just under the surface... What are you thinking about this goal?*

2. *Once you uncover your hidden beliefs, name them. Literally. So that when they come up you will quickly recognize them.* When you're on the way to exercise and that familiar laziness comes over you, say to yourself, "Oh, that's just my belief that life shouldn't be hard. Now how can I make this more fun?"

3. *When you have found your beliefs and named them, it's time to decide whether you want to keep them or get rid of them. After all, if you created a belief, you can get rid of it, too.* Your thoughts are your creations... just like stories in your mind. And your beliefs are simply thoughts you think over and over again.

4. *If there are some beliefs that you realize don't serve you, then you get to choose a new replacement belief.* Just remember that your brain will want to keep going back to the old belief. And you will just keep noticing when it does that and gently steer your mind to the new belief that feels much better. For example, in the health and exercise scenario, your new belief might be something like: life *is* short and I want to feel and be my best during this life I have.

5. And last, play a mental game with yourself. In order for the new belief to stick and feel natural, you need to *train yourself to look for evidence that the new belief is true.* So when you do get yourself to the gym, notice how great you

feel afterward, and consciously think: "I feel great! This was so worth it."

Eventually, your old beliefs will be history, and your new beliefs will support your goals and help you reach them faster than you thought possible.

Dive deeper into this concept. Do the exercise of the corresponding worksheet.

Worksheet 19: Uncover Your Beliefs That Conflict with Your Goals

It's a funny thing about our beliefs. Even if we're not completely aware of what they are, deep down, they hold the power to shape our lives. Right now, *who we are and what our life is like is directly related to those inner beliefs about what we think we're worth and what we think we can do.*

So it's time to dig up those secret beliefs that are holding us back and deal with them so we can stop sabotaging our efforts.

1. When you think about losing weight, and you have a plan, and you are excited, what lurks under the surface? **What are you telling yourself about your chances of succeeding? How do your past "failures" influence your ability to believe in yourself this time?**

_____

_____

_____

_____

2. Name these beliefs. If you always think that life is hard and weight loss is hard, it's obvious that these thoughts will hold you back. So name them. As in: the "My *life is hard* belief." Then when this comes up, you can recognize it and say, "Oh, that's just my old belief that life is too hard for this to work for me." and you can dismiss it and move on.

_____

_____

_____

_____

3. *You see what your secret beliefs are. You've named them so you can recognize them.* **Now you get to decide: keep or toss? If you keep it, make sure it feels good and moves you forward.** *If you want to toss a belief, you get to create a new one that does feel good and does move you forward.*

_____

_____

_____

_____

4. It's time to choose some new beliefs to replace the ones you decided to drop. So instead of thinking "poor me, I'm always so deprived. It's not fair," you might think, "I'm so lucky in so many ways."

_____

_____

_____

_____

5. And now look for evidence to prove this new belief right. For example, using "I'm so lucky in so many ways" evidence for this might be seeing that you have people in your life who love you. Or seeing that you are basically healthy. Or recognizing that you have the ability to make changes if you want to. It's all in your perspective.

_____

_____

_____

_____

What Went Wrong?

Are your goals achievable by you?

You set goals that don't make sense for you. You set goals that are not do-able, and in doing so, **you set yourself up for certain disappointment.**

Lesson 20: Setting Real Goals for Your Life and Your Body

Most of us are not masters at goal setting. We set them, mentally at least, and then are shocked that they don't actually happen. And we're not even talking about the action required to achieve goals....we're just talking about setting goals that are REAL for you... and actually achievable.

How do most of us set goals?

We make our goals unrealistic—We think

> *The reason most people never reach their goals is that they don't define them, or ever seriously consider them as believable or achievable.*
>
> *Winners can tell you where they are going, what they plan to do along the way, and who will be sharing the adventure with them.*
>
> ~Denis Watley

148

that when we lose weight we should look like a cross between a model and a movie star. We are totally disconnected from the reality of how we look and how we want to look.

We make our goals huge! When you have a goal like, say, to lose 107 pounds, or even 48 pounds, or even 23 pounds, this isn't something you can do in a day or a week or even a month. It's big. And it needs to be broken down. So when we have such a big goal and we take our first baby step, the size of the task ahead of us just shuts us down with a feeling of being overwhelmed.

We set goals that don't faintly resemble the life we live. Most of us won't do well if our goal requires that we have a personal trainer, a private chef, and a life coach on call 24/7. **We need to take our life into consideration and decide what would actually work for us.**

Our life

Our body.

Our reality.

Our mind.

Although all these things can be changed, we need to begin by working with what we've got. It has to be relevant to us. Not to the folks in the pages of *People Magazine*.

Why is this a much better way to set goals?

Because it's do-able. You will see results.

Your achievable results will act as stepping-stones to the *next* step.

And you'll really be doing it.

You'll get excited.

And then, you will see the results you've been looking for.

So how do you set these REAL goals?

You start with your big goal and first do a mental check:

> *Is this really achievable?*
>
> *By me?*
>
> *Do I know anyone who did this? Is it possible?*
>
> *How can I break it down?*
>
> *What would the tiniest step forward be? How will I measure my progress?*
>
> *How will I know when I've achieved it?*
>
> *What are some resting places along the way to my big goal where I can pause and assess my progress?*

So let's get started. Maybe in the past you haven't set goals that were realistic to your life. But now you will. That's the first step toward getting what you want.

Dive deeper into this concept. Go to the corresponding worksheet and do the exercise.

Worksheet 20: How to Set Real Goals

If you keep setting goals for yourself and not achieving them, part of the problem might be that your goals don't fit your life.

Choose a goal you really want, and **then use this checklist to determine if this goal is real, for your life, for your body, for you.**

1. My goal is: (What do you want to do, to be or to have?)

_____

_____

_____

_____

2. Is this achievable in the real world?

_____

_____

_____

_____

3. Do I know anyone who has actually achieved this goal?

_____

_____

_____

_____

4. If I can think of someone who did this, do I know how they did it?

_____

_____

_____

_____

5. Is this possible given my reality?

_____

_____

_____

_____

6. How can I break this goal down into actionable steps?

_____

_____

_____

_____

7. Do I need help?

_____

_____

_____

_____

8. What would my first step be?

_____

_____

_____

_____

9. How will I measure my progress?

_____

_____

_____

_____

10. How will I know when I've actually reached my goal?

_____

_____

_____

_____

11. What are some resting places along the way to my goal where I can pause, assess how I'm doing and what I need, and then move on?

_____

_____

_____

_____

12. What will I do to celebrate reaching my goal?

_____

_____

_____

_____

What Went Wrong?

Are you waiting until you lose weight to feel good?

You expect to feel great when you lose weight. But you have no ability to create good feelings for yourself now. So you feel terrible and expect that negative feeling to motivate you. This simply doesn't work.

Lesson 21: Feel Good First, Not When You Are at Your Dream Weight

---

Have you ever told yourself that you'll be happy when you lose weight?

When your kids do better in school?

When your husband earns more money?

Or when you finally have time to relax?

What we tell ourselves, our thoughts, are what create how we feel. So when we constantly tell ourselves that we will be happy when _____ happens, well, that doesn't create a really good-feeling present moment. It takes all responsibility away from us, and we believe our happiness depends on some outside event happening. So out of our control!

When we wait for our happiness in this way, we don't feel great. We think thoughts that create our negative moods. We might feel frustrated, sad, impatient with ourselves, or disappointed. When we have these types of uncomfortable feelings, we tend to take negative actions.

Like eat to get rid of these feelings. And get negative results. Like a weight gain. What a vicious cycle!

We think we can't be happy until something happens, and then we think so negatively that the thing we are waiting for and depending on doesn't happen!

This crazy cycle not only doesn't work... but it feels crappy.

What does work is this: feeling good right now.

What?

How can I feel good at this weight, you ask?

Feeling good at this weight is totally within your control. It's the ultimate inside job.

Because it comes from your thoughts.

Instead of thinking, "I'm so overweight. I'll never be thin," which makes you feel hopeless and helpless. Try thinking something like, "I'm in the process of taking care of myself and losing weight." For most of my clients, using a phrase like "I'm in the process" makes them feel hopeful and powerful.

When we have good feelings, we tend to take actions that bring us closer to what we want.

So the better our thoughts are, right now, the better we'll feel.

The better we feel, the better actions we'll take.

And the better actions we take on a consistent basis, the more we get the results we want.

So, getting back to weight loss... I know that when you begin a program, any program, you may be hopeful. And at the same time you may be at a low point emotionally.

Why a low point?

Because if you're like most women, this isn't the first time you've tried to lose weight. You're not new to this. And chances are you are judging yourself by your past failures.

Unfortunately, focusing on your past failures won't get you any closer to success. But learning how to create good feelings right now will.

Absolutely.

How can you do this?

Right now, I want you to know that you are here for a reason. You are starting a weight loss program at exactly the right time.

And everything you have learned about yourself from your past efforts will now come together and work for you, not against you.

All you have to do is take those lessons and keep moving ahead. With a good feeling.

Hopeful. Trusting yourself that you can do this. Confident that if anyone else in the world has resolved her weight issues, then you can too.

All those feelings come from powerful thoughts. And all those good feelings will help you take the right actions you need to stay on your program and move forward.

Finally!

So remember, you are in control. Let's dig up those good feelings now.

Dive deeper into this concept. Go to the corresponding worksheet and do the exercise.

Worksheet 21: How to Feel Good First

Remember back in lesson 14 how we uncovered the feelings you want? Well now it's time to figure out how to get some of those feelings now. The better you feel now, at your current weight, the easier it will be to take the actions that will get you to your natural weight.

Imagine trying to eat mindfully and change some habits while you feel hopeless, cranky, and resentful. My bet is that you won't get far on your program. Now imagine that even though your weight hasn't changed yet, you feel confident and optimistic. Any program you choose will be easier and smoother because of your good feelings.

So let's go back to the feelings you want to create...often I hear words like "confident, powerful, free, hopeful, optimistic, strong, and peaceful."

1. Take the first of your words describing how you'd like to feel:

_____

_____

_____

_____

2. What do you do right now in your life that gives you a similar feeling?

_____

_____

_____

_____

3. What can you do to get that feeling more often?

_____

_____

_____

_____

4. What can you *think* of to conjure that feeling up on a regular basis?

_____

_____

_____

_____

5. Can you think of a role model you know or even a public figure who seems to embody the feeling you want?

_____

_____

_____

_____

6. Imagine that you wake up one day and that feeling is now inside of you... What will your thinking be like?

_____

_____

_____

_____

7. Each day, choose how you want to feel and remember these steps to create that feeling right now.

_____

_____

_____

_____

8. Repeat this exercise with each of the words you chose to describe how you want to feel.

_____

_____

_____

_____

What Went Wrong?

Do you think what happens is out of your control?

You think things just happen to you. You aren't aware of the power you have in your own mind. You think if you could only change your circumstances, you'd be happier and lose more weight. But you don't know that **your thoughts are in charge of your happiness.**

Lesson 22: What Do Your Thoughts Have to Do with It?

If you've ever been unhappy, obviously you're not alone. Every single one of us has experienced a full range of positive and not-so-positive emotions. And usually, when we're miserable, we automatically go right to what we think is causing our unhappiness: our circumstances.

We think we're upset because our child got a D on her report card.

We're angry because we were promised a certain delivery date and the package never showed.

Or we feel rejected because our friend forgot our birthday.

> *Minds need cleaning at least as often as houses.*
>
> ~Brooke Castillo

And, let's not forget this one: we step on the scale and see that our weight has gone up, and now we feel hopeless and ashamed.

In all of these examples, **we're actually not unhappy because of what happened in our lives. We're unhappy because of what we're telling ourselves about it. We're unhappy because of our thoughts about it.**

When our child gets a D on her report card, we may think "I'm a lousy parent."

When our package doesn't show up on time, we may think "I have bad luck! I never get what I need on time!"

When our friend forgets our birthday, we might think "She doesn't care about me."

And when we step on the scale and see the numbers going up, we may think, "There must be something wrong with me!"

This concept is true even with good feelings.

We think we're in a great mood because we lost seven pounds. But actually, we're happy because we are thinking that means we are finally worthy.

We think we're proud because our child got into a special honors class. But actually we are proud because we're telling ourselves we did a great job as a parent.

Or we think we're happy because we have a certain amount of money in the bank, but the reality is that we are happy because we're telling ourselves this amount means we are safe and secure.

Can you see the difference?

It is never our circumstance that makes us happy or unhappy.

It's the story we tell ourselves about it that determines our feelings. This is important news when we're trying to lose weight.

If you are like many of my clients, maybe you eat when you are feeling an uncomfortable emotion.

And you tell yourself it's because something happened that made you feel uncomfortable.

Well, I have the best news for you... Your circumstances are just neutral. That's right. They are just facts.

It's your story about them, your thoughts that make you feel good or bad.

And the beautiful thing is that you can change your thoughts. Just like that.

And then you will change how you feel.

I learned this a few years ago from Brooke Castillo, who wrote the book *Self Coaching 101 – Use Your Mind – Don't Let It Use You.*

This opened up my eyes to a whole new world... a world in which I wasn't walking around with my fingers crossed hoping to have a good day.

It gave me back my power because I learned how to create thoughts that would help me get what I wanted most: to feel good.

When you feel good, you can accomplish most anything.

And when you don't feel good, you're at the mercy of what

happens in the world around you. And that is not such good news.

Your circumstance creates your thoughts. Your thoughts create your feelings.

Your feelings cause you to take certain actions.

And the actions you take create certain results for you.

So if you interrupt this chain and keep your circumstance the same, but change your thoughts about it, you will feel differently, take different actions, and voila! You will get a different result.

A result you choose.

This is a big topic.

But this is just a little taste of why you may have been overeating and gaining weight, even though you say you want to lose weight.

Your thoughts are the main ingredient.

Look at how you feel, and then look at what you are thinking. If you change the thought, you will feel differently.

And with good feelings, your whole life can be different.

Dive deeper into this concept. Go to the corresponding worksheet and do the exercise.

Worksheet 22: Working on Your Thoughts

(Self-coaching model created by Brooke Castillo)

Now you have a basic understanding of how your thoughts create your feelings, which lead you to take actions, and those actions give you results in your life. This is a deep subject, but for starters, I'd like you to see the process in action and realize that you are in charge of your thoughts. And if you're not happy with the way you feel emotionally, or the actions you take, or the results you have, then it's time to look at your thoughts and morph them into thoughts that are better for you, all the way down the chain of events (thought, feeling, action, result).

1. What is the circumstance?

_____

_____

_____

_____

2. What thought does the circumstance trigger?

_____

_____

_____

_____

3. What do you feel when you think this thought?

_____

_____

_____

_____

4. How do you act when you feel this way?

_____

_____

_____

_____

5. What is the result of this action?

_____

_____

_____

_____

6. How does the result prove the original thought?

_____

_____

_____

_____

7. What is a better-feeling thought to choose concerning this circumstance?

_____

_____

_____

_____

Do this model for every thought you have that leads to a negative feeling, and see what you can create in your life.

What Went Wrong?

Do you focus on what you don't want, instead of what you want?

Your focus is all over the place. You pay attention to what you don't want more than to what you do want. You don't realize the power that your focus has to bring you closer or further from what you're looking for.

Lesson 23: Focus Changes Everything

If you've ever watched the *Oprah* show in the last decade, no doubt you've heard the phrase "Law of Attraction." Today you're going to learn exactly what it is and how it applies to your weight loss.

The Law of Attraction is a concept that states that "like attracts like"...that we attract to ourselves what we feel, what we believe and what we focus on.

Does that mean that we always cause everything that happens to us in life? No, there are other forces and randomness to the universe that take credit for some things. Genetic accidents and lifestyle might account for who gets sick and who doesn't.

Location on the planet might account for earthquakes and floods. And imagine how many factors might play into the ups and downs of the stock market.

But in our own lives, there are certain things that come to us, or don't come to us that we *can* control.

And one of the factors affecting your weight loss is indeed the Law of Attraction. It's what you tell yourself *and* what you really believe that will determine what you focus on. And if you focus on something, and it feels good and you really believe it's possible, it will be easy for you to take actions that will take you closer to your weight loss goal.

If you want to lose weight, but secretly, or not so secretly don't believe you can, or don't believe it's possible, your beliefs will become a self-fulfilling prophesy. And you won't lose weight.

So don't just say, "I'm going to lose twenty-five pounds. I can do it!" without really believing you can. Look for evidence that you can. Cultivate the belief that you can.

Don't focus on your extra weight. Don't think about how "fat" you are. That will bring a feeling of defeat... You will keep doing what you've always done, and what will you get? More weight. **Focus on what you want, not on what you don't want.**

When you catch yourself focusing on what you *don't* like about your body, quickly redirect your thoughts to what you *do* like.

You aren't lying to yourself... You are just focusing on something you're not in the habit of focusing on.

In the end, you do have to take actions to lose weight, no doubt about it.

But it will be easier to take actions if you believe you can.

And if you can envision yourself doing it.

Belief first. Then focus.

Then comes the evidence.

As Wayne Dyer says, "You'll see it when you believe it, NOT you'll believe it when you see it."

Dive deeper into this concept. Go to the corresponding worksheet and do the exercise.

Worksheet 23: Learn How to Control Your Focus

Research on the way our brains function shows that *when it comes to good things, our minds are like Teflon.* We think about them briefly and then we quickly focus on something else.

And we process negative things more like Velcro. These negative thoughts stick around a lot longer and are harder to get rid of.

We are hardwired to focus on the negative for survival reasons, yet if we focus on what we don't want, or on what doesn't feel good, we will get more of exactly that. Our goal is to keep returning our focus to the positive, on what we do want.

Here are some ways to be mindful of where your focus is, and to train yourself to keep returning it to what you really want:

1. Each day, set an intention in the morning. How do you want to feel today? How do you want your day to go? Whatever it is you are working on, you are giving your mind instructions on where you want it to focus.

_____

_____

_____

_____

2. As your day continues, and you move into different segments, like getting to work, going to a meeting, coming home, starting to cook dinner... **pause briefly and set your intentions for each segment of your day.** By noticing and asking how you want things to go, you are directing your focus, instead of allowing your old brain wiring to take you right to the negative.

_____

_____

_____

_____

3. When your mind asks a negative question, leading to other negative thoughts, jump in and turn it into a positive question. This question should make you stimulated and excited. For example: I don't have time to shop and prep food for myself. That takes you down the road to all the reasons you can't do this. Ask yourself: How can I make time to shop for and prep food for myself? This will get your mind focused in the right direction on solutions and possibilities.

_____

_____

_____

_____

4. Notice when your mind goes to a negative spin. Name it. Say, "Oops, there I go into the negative. That's just the way my brain is wired. Let me change my focus."

_____

_____

_____

_____

5. Create some visual reminders that you will see periodically during the day. Post its. Calendar notes. Favorite sayings on your desktop of your computer. Keep bringing your mind back to the positive.

_____

_____

_____

_____

6. Use your feelings as a guide to let you know when your focus is slipping. As soon as you start to feel down in any way, that's a signal that your thoughts are going back to the negative. Catch them and pop your focus back to what feels good and what you want.

_____

_____

_____

_____

What Went Wrong?

Do you think about what's wrong instead of what's right?

You constantly think about what isn't going well. What you did wrong. Any misstep you made. You pretty much ignore anything you did that was right, went well, and took you a step closer to your goals. *You are negating the good things you are doing simply because you're still not there yet.*

Lesson 24: What Are You Doing Right?

It used to be that when I asked my clients how they were and how they had been doing, I'd get a long laundry list of all the things they thought they had done wrong.

> *-I had a binge last night and feel terrible today.*

> *-I got so upset with my husband that I finished a big bag of potato chips last week.*

> *-You wouldn't believe how little exercise I've done since we spoke.*

And on and on.

You'd think there was some big benefit to focusing on what they did wrong!

Literally!

I'd bet that if I called you and asked you the same question, and we were talking about your weight loss efforts, the first thing you'd focus on were the things you thought were not going well.

When we focus on what is wrong with us, our life, our bodies, our actions... the thoughts created from this negative spotlight make us feel bad.

Ashamed.

Hopeless.

Depressed.

And fundamentally flawed.

So what happens then?

Well, when we feel bad, we tend to take actions that aren't in our best interests. We focus on the negative, which causes negative feelings, and then we take negative actions.

So why are we surprised when we get negative results?

Well, after realizing how commonplace this was, I now have a new way to check in with my clients, and you should adopt this too.

The first question I ask them, and I train them to ask themselves, is "What am I doing right?"

Every day.

A lot of us are in the habit, or should be, of doing a daily gratitude list. In your head or on paper, thinking of what we are grateful for puts our brains in a place of peace and we are able to receive even more in our lives.

Well, after you pay attention to what you are grateful for, it's my strong suggestion that you then focus on what you've done right.

Think of it as a daily boast.

You did it when you were a kid, remember?

We'd come back to school after a weekend or a holiday break and couldn't wait to raise our hand to share with our teacher and our class what we had done that felt good.

We weren't modest about it.

I mean, we could really brag.

And bragging made us feel good.

So here's the deal. When you are trying to lose weight, you are going to take a series of steps. Some will "take" right away. Some will be more challenging and will have to be repeated numerous times. But if you have been focusing on what went wrong instead of what went right, it's no wonder you weren't as successful as you would have liked.

Some of us think that boasting means we are self-centered. Too full of ourselves.

But when we think about what is right, we create good feelings. And that is the only route to what you want... continued success on the road to permanent weight loss.

It's also a way of caring for ourselves... and getting our needs met, so we can give more of our gifts to the world.

Not at all self-centered in my book.

So think of this as a daily practice. Perhaps at the end of your day.

Ask: What did I do right today? And literally list every little thing. Say it out loud.
And notice how good you feel. Proud. Happy.

Capable. Optimistic. And when you feel this way,

you will follow with more good actions.

I promise.

And by the way, no need to list what you did wrong.

You probably already spend way too much time going over that list in your head. Think of those things that you could have done better as stepping stones in the school of life.

And get right back to the "what I did right" list.

Dive deeper into this concept. Go to the corresponding worksheet and do the exercise.

Worksheet 24: Focus on What You Are Doing Right

When I ask my clients how they are doing, I usually hear a list of everything they think has gone wrong. Everything they think they should have done better. And by the time they're finished, they feel awful and hopeless and I feel sympathetically exhausted. So I train them to first **focus on what is going well**. What they have done that they feel good about. This creates much better feelings... hopeful, proud, and confident. Then we can tackle what hasn't gone well with strength. Make sense?

I want to you start here and *keep an ongoing list of every little thing you are doing that takes you in the right direction.* You will be amazed at how this little shift in focus will make you feel better. And when you feel good, you will take actions that are positively inspired.

What am I doing right? What's going well? What am I proud of?

Keep going... train yourself to always focus on the positive first.

1.

2.

3.

4.

5.

6.

7.

8.

9.

10

11.

12.

13.

14.

15.

16.

17.

18.

19.

20.

21.

22.

23.

24.

25.

26.

27

28.

29.

30.

31.

32.

33.

34.

35.

36.

37.

38.

39.

40.

What Went Wrong?

Are you stuck in a comfortable rut?

You stay in your safe little comfort zone. You want to keep doing what you've always done, yet you expect to miraculously get a different result.

Lesson 25: Why You Need to Get Out of Your Comfort Zone!

━━━━━━━━━━━━━━━━━━━━━━━━━━━━━━━━━━━━━━

Today's lesson will make you uncomfortable. I hope. Let me explain.

Most of us operate smack in the middle of our comfort zone. **Our comfort zone is a state of security and low risk. It's where we spend most of our time, repeating the patterns and routines of doing the same things over and over again.**

This zone isn't all bad. It keeps us comfortable with low levels of stress and anxiety. It's where life is predictable.

We need to have a comfort zone. If we don't, we'll have *too much* stress and anxiety. We won't be able to function comfortably.

But if we keep our comfort zone too small, boredom sets in.

Too small, no good.

Too big, no good.

But **when your comfort zone is just right, it feels just great. You do just the right amount of things that make you stretch, just enough.** You feel a little anxiety but it's "optimal anxiety," just enough to get you to take some risks that will get you what you want most.

The fact is that although staying in our comfort zone is, well, comfy, we need that stretch to keep expanding it... We need the challenge to reach our peak.

When you want to lose weight, you've got to find that delicate balance between never pushing yourself, and throwing out everything you've always done and starting fresh.

You don't have to go to either extreme... but you do need to figure out where you are, *and* where you want to go.

And then choose a goal that scares you. Just a little.

Not something that scares you so much you want to jump back in bed and pull the covers over your head.

But something that you truly think is doable... and maybe you don't know the "how" part yet.

Something that feels awkward but promises you a sweet reward.

Stepping out of your comfort zone has a major reward, by the way.

By doing something that pushes you beyond your own mental blocks, you are now enlarging your comfort zone.

And in the future you'll now be able to do more. With no stress. So what do you wish you could do to take care of yourself?

To move your body?

To have delicious, healthy food available?

Don't look at what you've always done. Look at options outside of your usual repertoire.

And then take a leap.

Get support if you need it. But take a leap and have faith in yourself.

Even if you fall, you'll learn something and be able to take a bigger step next time.

So think about it. What is holding you back from doing something you know would make a difference in your life?

And now find a way to do it. It's ok to be afraid.

But it's not okay to let fear keep you locked in that tight, cramped little zone of comfort.

Dive deeper into this concept. Go to the corresponding worksheet and do the exercise.

Worksheet 25: How to Get Out of Your Comfort Zone

There's something you want very much. But whenever you think of doing what you need to do to get there, you get a funny feeling in the pit of your stomach. You think you can't do it because you've never done it before. And it might be a tad uncomfortable.

Your comfort zone, while comfy, keeps you right where you are. And when you push through it in a smart way, you'll enlarge that zone where you feel comfortable and confident. So let's go... no more staying where you are!

1. You want to do something... (Fill in what you long to do.)

_____

_____

_____

_____

2. You feel discomfort: specifically, you feel:

_____

_____

_____

_____

3. What are you telling yourself that causes that feeling:

_____

_____

_____

_____

4. Imagine if you could gently push yourself through your comfort zone in this area and do what you want to do. What would it look like?

_____

_____

_____

_____

5. How would you feel if you could do this?

_____

_____

_____

_____

6. What would you be thinking?

_____

_____

_____

_____

I'd like you to view the border of your comfort zone as the place where you are holding yourself back. It's not a brick wall. _Think of it as an escalator_ that you can get on to go to the next level. Or not.

7. What's the smallest action you can take to go through your comfort zone toward what you want?

_____

_____

_____

_____

Now take that small action. Get on that escalator. And congratulate yourself! You've just enlarged your comfort zone!

What Went Wrong?

Are you waiting to be in the mood to take action?

You wait to feel inspired before you take action. **You think you need to be "in the mood" to do something.** You don't realize the value of taking action and getting inspired from that action.

Lesson 26: Take Action to Ignite Inspiration

In Lesson 21, you learned how important it was to feel good first, even before you achieve your goal. And in lesson 22, you learned how your thoughts create the feelings you experience. And how those feelings lead you to take action.

All of that is true. And valuable information.

But there is one more life-changing perspective that can help you on this journey and here it is:

Sometimes you need to take action first.

Before you have worked on your thoughts and your feelings.

> *Taking action is the only way to start the path to realizing your dreams... Take a first step towards that goal and see how the universe backs you up.*
>
> ~Carmen Marie

Before you feel inspired. Even if you don't feel like it.

Because when you take action, you are giving yourself evidence that you can do something.

And then your thoughts and beliefs will follow. Let me give you an example:

You have a great idea for a book.

You want to write it and get it out into the world because you know people would benefit from your ideas.

Day after day you sit at your desk waiting to be inspired to write.

And nothing comes.

Nothing.

But one day you take yourself by the hand and push yourself to write one page.

Just one little page. And you do it.

And guess what?

You feel proud. Excited! More confident.

What was an overwhelming task and huge dream is suddenly feeling more possible.

Why? Because that one page you wrote gave you evidence that you could do it.

Sometimes if you sit around waiting to get aligned with your thoughts and your feelings, a long time can pass before you actually do something.

So sometimes, you just need to take action.

It's like working backward, but it works.

Are you waiting to get in the mood to sit down and plan your grocery list for the week, so you'll have delicious food available?

Just sit down and do it.

Are you waiting to get in the mood to walk around the block? Don't wait for the mood. Create the mood by getting on your shoes and getting out the door.

There is something to be said for the great Nike slogan... *Just Do It.*

Try to create a feeling that will make it easy for you to lace up those gym shoes.

But if you've tried and it's not happening, then get off your butt and just do it.

And the inspiration will come.

Dive deeper into this concept. Go to the corresponding worksheet and do the exercise.

Worksheet 26: Learn to Take Action to Create Inspiration

You know that if you sit around and wait until a certain mood comes to you before you do something, you might be sitting around for a very long time. The trick is to clean up your thoughts and feel good enough to take action. But sometimes even when we do that, it still feels like lifting a large boulder. So we procrastinate.

And procrastinate. And procrastinate.

And then, we have to do what Nike tells us: Just Do It!

We have to take a small action. That action will make us feel different. Usually much better. And with that more positive feeling, taking the next action will be easier. And on and on and on.

Here's what it looks like with an example from Lesson 26.

Your goal: to write a book

Your obstacle: you can't get started. You are procrastinating.

Your mood: helpless, overwhelmed

The smallest action you can take: write for fifteen minutes

Your new feeling after taking it: proud, competent, and excited

Your next action: write again for a slightly longer time... and celebrate!

Now it's your turn.

Think of something you are trying to get yourself to do in the world of weight loss. Move your body? Prepare a nice meal for yourself? Slow down enough to look at your thoughts?

1. Your goal:

_____

_____

_____

_____

2. Your obstacle:

_____

_____

_____

_____

3. Your mood:

_____

_____

_____

_____

4. The smallest action you can take:

_____

_____

_____

_____

5. Your new feeling after taking it:

_____

_____

_____

_____

6. Your next action:

_____

_____

_____

_____

Now go and do it! One tiny thing.

What Went Wrong?

Are you underestimating the importance of all your choices?

You make small choices that take you off course. And you tell yourself that it's no big deal. It's better than it used to be. And maybe it is. But you are forgetting that **every single choice you make counts.** And takes you in a direction that is either further away or closer to your desired end.

Lesson 27: Every Choice Counts

Does this sound familiar?

-Oh, it's just one bite! It's no big deal!

-I'll just start my eating plan tomorrow.

-I'm so tired; I can exercise next week.

-That was so delicious; I'll have another helping.

If this sounds like some of the things you've thought or said before, you're not alone. Taken one at a time, each of these situations sounds unimportant. And they are...not a big deal. But added up over time, they compound...just like interest in a savings account.

All the minute choices you make, day in and day out, all add up eventually. And they give you the results you now have in your life.

Every extra pound on your body is a result of thousands of tiny choices that added up to big results.

We might not like our current results, our current weight, or our current body. But let's take the mystery out of it. There is nothing wrong with you. And there is nothing wrong with your life.

You've made certain choices and over time, they've given you what you have now. In all areas of your life.

These choices, in the moment they are presented to us, seem small. Totally inconsequential.

So as easy as it is to eat that piece of fruit, it's also easy to not do it.

As easy as it is to check to see if you are hungry, it's such a small thing that it's also easy to just not do.

And, as easy as it is to just say "no" to a second helping of something delicious, in that moment, it's also easy to not say "no" to the second helping.

Jeff Olson writes about how these choices add up in his great book, *The Slight Edge.* I apply this concept to my life, my work, and my coaching programs.

Easy to do.

And easy to not do.

Awareness is the key here.

And the knowledge that every single thing you do will have a consequence.

So be present.

And be honest with yourself. Stop saying it's no big deal.

It may not be a big deal, but when you do something 793 times, it is a big deal, and it does count.

It all counts.

Dive deeper into this concept. Go to the corresponding worksheet and do the exercise.

Worksheet 27: Make Every Choice Count

"Every choice counts. Choose wisely." Don Shapiro

Every single thing you do or don't do every day counts. Each choice leads you to your next choice. And *influences* that next choice. And they all add up. To the results you create each day, each week, each month and each year. *And this is what makes up your life.*

So if you're less than thrilled with your current life or habits or body, it's time to slow down and look at every choice you make. Be conscious because it all makes a difference.

Take a look at the sequence of events of this first day, and see how each choice led to the next choice:

Day 1:

1. Woke up late

2. Skipped breakfast

3. Grabbed a coffee and pastry from the cart at work

4. Felt tired soon after eating, didn't get a lot done

5. Blood sugar so low ate a candy bar from vending machine to stay awake

6. Felt sluggish, needed to work through part of lunch

7. Went to fast food drive-through for lunch and ate in the car

8. Felt down, and thought "I've blown it today"

9. Had another candy bar in the afternoon to keep going

10 Got home late, was too tired to cook, ordered in pizza

11. Vegged out in front of the television and overate

12. Felt depressed and pessimistic, vowed to do better tomorrow

13. Fell asleep on the couch and forgot to set the alarm

14. Repeated the same pattern the next day

Now take a look at another day where one positive choice led to another and another:

Day 2:

1. Woke up late (a negative start, right? But here you made a U-turn)

2. Grabbed a protein bar and some bottled water on the way to work

3. Had coffee and more water when you got to work

4. Worked hard, took breaks, and felt productive

5. Had a delicious restaurant lunch with a friend

6. Worked industriously through the afternoon

7. Took an afternoon break and had some fruit, nuts, and tea

8. During break, you planned your dinner menu

9. Walked home using the gym shoes you carried in your tote bag

10. Got home and changed clothes, played with your pet

11. Cooked a delicious, easy dinner while listening to music

12. Indulged in "me" time, reading, thinking, planning

13. Set alarm so you would be on time tomorrow

Now it's your turn. *Think of a recent day where one bad choice let to a generally not-great day.*

And then create a great day, either one you had or one you want to have, where each mostly positive choice led to the next positive choice.

And remember, if you don't make a choice that is taking you where you want to go, just make a U-turn and either redo your choice, or make up for it the very next opportunity you have.

Your not-great day:

     1.

     2.

     3.

     4.

     5.

     6.

     7.

     8.

     9.

     10.

Your real or potentially real great day:

     1.

     2.

     3.

     4.

     5.

     6.

     7.

     8.

     9.

     10.

What Went Wrong?

Do you set goals and then forget them?

You set goals and then you get distracted. You literally forget that you were working on something. You wake up and time has passed and you've lost your focus. *You haven't created a plan to keep your goals in front of you.*

Lesson 28: How to Keep Your Goals on the Front Burner

Here we are on the subject of goals again. Why are we so goal-oriented? Because if you want to lose your extra weight for good, you need to focus on what you want. And having very specific goals is part of what will get you there.

But one problem that many of my clients run into is this: they set a goal, they map out all the action steps they will have to take, and then, poof! They forget all about it!

The craziness of daily life takes over. We get busy. We get phone calls and emails and urgent requests.

So we disconnect from the big picture of what we want and we focus on what is calling for our immediate attention.

Sometimes we do need to be flexible and responsive to what is happening in front of us. But if we continually do this at our own expense, we will never be able to really make changes.

And the sad thing is, we blame ourselves.

Nothing is wrong here. It's just that you forgot one big step.

Set some reminders to keep your goals and the next steps you need to take on the front burner of your mind.

We need to remind ourselves to check in and look at our goals, look at our next steps and figure out when we will do them.

Every day.

This is not a set-it-and-forget-it deal.

So many women sign up for a weight loss program and are really excited. That's good. But sometimes it stops there.

Their excitement from signing up isn't enough to get them through it. They actually have to take steps.

And before they take any steps, they have to *remember* to check in and see what's next.

So make a plan. A routine. A daily ritual.

For example, every morning you could look at your list and make sure that some things related to your goals are on it.

Then you need to figure out where in your day or night you will do them.

And then, set some physical reminders.

A computer reminder system might work if you are at a desk all day long.

You can set phone reminders to beep or vibrate when you want to prompt yourself to do something. You can even label it to tell yourself exactly what to do.

You can set up your digital calendar to tell you when it's time to do something for yourself.

Everything you've ever done to be on time, or to remember something for work, or for your family, can be used in your person goal program.

Purely to help you stay on track and keep taking actions.

The actions aren't so hard.

It's just getting yourself to remember what to do next.

You can do this!

What's a simple daily ritual you can set up for yourself to remind you of the next personal action you want to take?

Dive deeper into this concept. Go to the corresponding worksheet and do the exercise.

Worksheet 28: Keeping Your Goals on the Front Burner

Have you ever worked on a big project? One that had many moving parts, lots of details, and many categories?

Well, losing weight and changing from the inside out is like working on a big project. And you are that project.

So when you plan a wedding, build a house, raise a child, or start a business, you wouldn't just get an idea and then sit back and expect things to start rolling until you were done. You'd plan. You'd set deadlines. You'd make lists. And you'd mark your calendar with reminders. After all, this project is pretty important.

I'm sure you can see where this is going. You are the most important thing in your life. It all starts with you. *So treating your weight loss as a project is something that will move you toward success.* This doesn't mean you need to plan every inch of your day or your life. But if you want something to happen, you have to help it happen. Get it organized. And set yourself up to remember what you need to do. It's so worth it. But it won't happen on its own. So let's get going on Project You.

1. Look at the big picture first... What has to happen *this month* in order to have what you need to eat well and move your body? Do you need to shop? Prep food? Research some recipes? Find a walking buddy? Block out time to think, or journal? Start with a list.

_____

_____

_____

_____

2. Let's make it a step more real: pull out your calendar and **plot out when you will do these things.** Mark them in ink.

_____

_____

_____

_____

3. Now we get down to looking at your week. On a Saturday or Sunday, **plan the coming week**. Make sure you are first on your list. Even if you care for an elderly person or a newborn, you need to be fed and rested so you have the energy to care for them. No excuses. Figure out what you need and how much time you need to care for yourself.

_____

_____

_____

_____

4. Let's look at your day. You already know what your week looks like...now, at the end of each day, take a peek at what's in store for tomorrow. How will you remember that you planned to cut up veggies and cook rice for the week? It's on your list. It's on your calendar. But how will you remember to look at the list or calendar? **Set a reminder**. Set your computer, kitchen oven clock, or cell phone alarm to go off and remind you. Just like you have an appointment.

_____

_____

_____

_____

You need to give yourself the best shot at making things happen. Not by accident. Not if you happen to remember. But on purpose. *Put it on the front burner of your mind and figure out what you need to do to keep it there.*

What Went Wrong?

Do you expect immediate results?

When you don't get immediate results, you stop. *You give up way too soon.* You follow a plan for three days and are discouraged when you don't see a major result. You take the short view, instead of the long view.

Lesson 29: Want Change? Take the Long View.

Whether the goal is to lose weight, get a promotion, or save a million dollars, some people will succeed and some will fail.

Do you know what the greatest cause of failure is?

It's quitting. Giving up.

And why do so many of us quit?

Because we are used to things happening instantaneously. And when they don't, we stomp our feet and walk away.

This is too hard. I just can't do it anymore. I tried... for a week, and it didn't work.

Sound familiar?

In our fast-moving world, we may be so used to everything happening ridiculously fast that when results are a little slower to show up, we give up.

But here's the thing: if you are trying to lose weight, the things you must do definitely take time. They're not instant.

The reality is that change occurs when we take small consistent actions over a long period of time.

Read that again. Really.

It can be boring. It may not be what you want to hear. But until you digest this reality, any change you attempt will not happen fast enough for you. And sadly, you will quit.

It's a little like planting a seed. You dig your hole and put the seed in the ground, covering it with soil filled with nutrients. You water it and wait. Finally it breaks the ground.

If you treated planting the seed the same way you treat undertaking a major life change, you might quickly get impatient. And dig up the seed and throw it away.

That's what we do when we embark on a change that takes time.

We argue with reality when we don't give it the time it needs to give us the results we want.

You are that seed.

You want to make big changes that will give you freedom from overeating and extra weight.

It's like you are planted and waiting to develop into who you want to be... a new you with new habits.

You are germinating.

Your results are in process.

But you must give it time.

Don't quit before you have a chance to see your results.

Don't give up too soon.

Dive deeper into this concept. Go to the corresponding worksheet and do the exercise.

Worksheet 29: How to Take the Long View for Change

You may give lip service to this concept, but it requires more than that. **Change does take time. And if we don't accept that truth, we do ourselves the deepest disservice: we quit too soon.**

Small actions.

With great consistency. Over the long haul.

To get the results we want.

Here's the formula:

> 1. You *start working your plan to* get the results you want, in any area of your life, and especially in your plan for weight loss.
>
> 2. You work the plan and *get results*.
>
> 3. *You* use these results as feedback.

4. You keep taking action and *testing new actions*.

5. You keep using your results as feedback.

6. You *experiment* to make the process feel as good as possible.

7. And you keep using your feedback.

8. Along the way you *give yourself rewards* for reaching milestones, and for staying on your path.

9. You get where you want to go. Whoo hoo!

10. You celebrate!

Success in 10 steps sounds simple but some things can and do take a lot of time. *If you have 30 or 50 or 100 pounds to lose, it might take a very long time. That is okay. That time will pass whether you reach your goal or not. So use the time to stay on your path.* It will be worth it, I promise.

Your Plan:

1. What's your general plan and what is your first step?

_____

_____

_____

_____

2. After you took a step, what result did you get?

_____

_____

_____

_____

3. Based on that result, do you keep going or adjust your course?

_____

_____

_____

_____

4. Continue to move forward.

_____

_____

_____

_____

5. Continue to evaluate your actions, based on the feedback you are getting.

_____

_____

_____

_____

6. Experiment a little, looking for ease and fun as you move forward.

_____

_____

_____

_____

7. Keep tracking your feedback. Is it working? Any adjustments needed?

_____

_____

_____

_____

8. What can you reward yourself with?

_____

_____

_____

_____

9. You are there! How does it feel?

_____

_____

_____

_____

10. Celebrate!!

_____

_____

_____

_____

Think of yourself as a peaceful warrior... You know what you want and you will do what it takes to get it. This is your mission. Just keep moving forward.

What Went Wrong?

Are you afraid to believe in yourself?

You are afraid to have hope. You have lost faith in yourself and halfheartedly try something while secretly believing it won't work for you. You look at others creating what you want, and don't realize that **what someone else can do, you can too.**

Lesson 30: Take a Leap of Faith

> *Things can fall apart, or threaten to, and then there's got to be a leap of faith.*
>
> *Ultimately, when you're at the edge, you have to go forward or backward; If you go forward, you have to jump together.*
>
> ~Yo-Yo Ma

All the little things you've learned in these lessons will serve you well as you continue on your path to eating and living like a naturally slim person.

All the small changes in perspective will add up, resulting in you looking at yourself, your efforts and your goals in a new way... if you practice them. So what's left for you to learn?

You need to learn to trust yourself.

To give yourself credit.

To believe in hope and possibility.

Here's the thing: there is nothing wrong with you. And there is nothing "special" about people who have tried to lose weight and succeeded.

In this world, anything that has been done by anyone else can be done by you. In a version that fits your life.

Maybe your body isn't happy running marathons. But there is a version of moving your body that would feel good.

Maybe your brain wouldn't be happy tracking what you eat and planning ahead, but I guarantee that there is a version of those strategies that would work for you.

So the key is knowing that if someone else did what you strive for, it can be done.

You just need to find your own personal path and begin.

Just begin.

Take a leap of faith in yourself, and know that you are capable of great things. No matter how many times you have failed in the past.

Stop using your tired, old excuses for why you can never lose weight, and start seeing possibility instead of brick walls.

It only takes one time to get it right. You *can* do this.

Dive deeper into this concept. Go to the corresponding worksheet and do the exercise.

Worksheet 30: How to Take a Leap of Faith

Life is an adventure, and your weight loss journey will be part of that adventure. Maybe it won't be a straight line to the end, but you will learn and grow and expand in ways you never dreamt of while on this journey.

So it's time to take what you've learned and make the leap from thinking you just can't do this, to having faith that you *can* do this.

In your life, not everything has come about in an easy way. Weight loss is no different. Even if you've struggled for years, you can still do this. I know this is true. **You are not an exception.**

Let's make it a no-brainer that you have a strong belief in yourself before you leap:

1. What good choices have you made in your life?

_____

_____

_____

_____

2. What have you worked hard for and achieved?

_____

_____

_____

_____

3. How do you know you can trust yourself?

_____

_____

_____

_____

4. What have you done that took multiple tries? And perhaps going back to the drawing board?

_____

_____

_____

_____

5. What are some qualities you have that make you proud?

_____

_____

_____

_____

6. What life lessons have you learned so far from all your efforts?

_____

_____

_____

_____

Are you ready? Starting now, you have a clean slate. You deserve this. Now take that leap.

About the Author

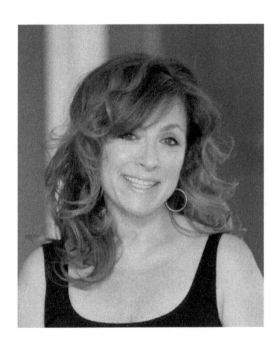

Cookie Rosenblum, M.A. is a life coach with only one specialty: Weight Loss. She is a Certified Life Coach through Martha Beck, PhD (known as Oprah's favorite life coach), and a Master Certified Coach through Brooke

Castillo, owner of The Life Coach School. Cookie has a master's degree in Clinical Psychology and uses a combination of coaching, psychology, and brain science to help her clients learn to think the way naturally thin people think.

Since 1986, Cookie has been helping smart women not only lose their extra weight, but also teaching them how to lose the whole problem. Her specialties are habitual overeating, emotional eating, and binge eating.

She works with groups and individuals both nationally and locally. Please contact Cookie at cookie@realweightlossrealwomen.com with any questions, comments, or suggestions you have regarding this book. Or, you can schedule a free consultation to see whether you might be interested in working with Cookie by emailing her at the email address above.

If you'd like to learn more about Cookie's programs, visit her at www.RealWeightLossRealWomen.com

Cookie's given name is Bettejane, but was nicknamed Cookie as a bald baby with a big, round face like a cookie. It's funny how things turn out!

She currently lives with her husband and two daughters in Indiana after spending most of her life in New York City and Chicago.

CPSIA information can be obtained
at www.ICGtesting.com
Printed in the USA
BVHW041138150322
631527BV00012B/256